COPING WITH

An Organ
Transplant

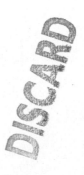

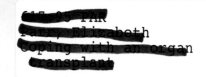

COPING WITH
An Organ
Transplant

A Practical Guide to Understanding, Preparing for, and Living with an Organ Transplant

ELIZABETH PARR, PH.D., and
JANET MIZE, R.N., CCTC

Avery
A MEMBER OF
PENGUIN PUTNAM INC.
NEW YORK

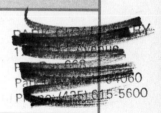

Every effort has been made to ensure that the information contained in this book is complete and accurate. However, neither the publisher nor the author is engaged in rendering professional advice or services to the individual reader. The ideas, procedures, and suggestions contained herein are not intended as a substitute for consulting with a physician. All matters regarding health require medical supervision. Neither the author nor the publisher shall be liable or responsible for any loss, injury or damage allegedly arising from any information or suggestion in this book.

Most Avery books are available at special quantity discounts for bulk purchase for sales promotions, premiums, fund-raising, and educational needs. Special books or book excerpts also can be created to fit specific needs. For details, write Putnam Special Markets, 375 Hudson Street, New York, NY 10014.

AVERY

a member of
Penguin Putnam Inc.
375 Hudson Street
New York, NY 10014
www.penguinputnam.com

Library of Congress Cataloging-in-Publication Data

Parr, Elizabeth.
Coping with an organ transplant : a practical guide to
understanding, preparing for, and living with an organ transplant /
Elizabeth Parr and Janet Mize.
p.   cm.
Includes bibliographical references and index.
ISBN 1-58333-092-5
1. Transplantation of organs, tissues, etc.   2. Consumer education.
I. Mize, Janet.   II. Title.
RD120.7 .P365   2001   00-069997
617.9'5—dc21

Printed in the United States of America
1   3   5   7   9   10   8   6   4   2

Book design by Jennifer Ann Daddio

Contents

PART THREE
Post-Transplant

Foreword

No field of medicine has benefited more from advances in technology than solid organ transplantation. Although the first successful renal transplant was performed by Dr. Joseph Murray in 1954, it was the introduction of the immunosuppressant cyclosporine in the late 1970s that increased one-year transplant survival from 10 percent to over 80 percent. Currently, the one-year patient survival rate for liver transplants approaches 80 percent and for cardiac transplantation, 90 percent. Similary, one-year graft survival for renal transplantation approaches 95 percent in many centers.

The tremendous success in cardiac, renal, and liver transplantation has resulted in an increased number of patients being referred for transplant evaluation. As a result, waiting times have dramatically lengthened, and more patients die while awaiting potentially life-saving operations. The waiting time disparities have generated a movement by the federal government to reorganize the organ allocation system (first with livers, then with other organs). However, what is lost in the debate is the fact that increasing the consent rate of potential organ donors would have a far greater impact on wait times.

When I first meet a potential organ transplant recipient, I always emphasize that the patient's entire "family" will be receiving the transplant. Without a strong social support system no patient could make it to, much less through, the transplant procedure. Although many transplant programs offer support groups for patient and family, until now there has been no "how-to" book for these individuals.

In this book Elizabeth Parr, Ph.D., and Janet Mize, R.N., CCTC, attempt to demystify the pretransplant, operative, and posttransplant regimens. They provide unique insight from the point of view of patient, coordinator, and primary caregiver. As experts in the field, they can describe firsthand the physical, mental, and emotional ups and downs associated with the disease process and the ultimate cure. Given the wealth and practicality of information provided, perhaps this book's title might have been *The Survivalist Guide to Transplantation.*

As you and your loved one embark on this journey, remember that this is a marathon, not a sprint. The short-term sacrifices will be great but the long-term rewards countless. On behalf of the transplant community, I wish you the best of luck in your adventure.

—David Imagawa, M.D., Ph.D.
Chief, Division of Transplantation
University of California-Irvine
Medical Center

Preface

When Elizabeth approached me with the idea of writing a book about the transplant process, I instantly saw a way to answer my own dilemma; getting out the true word about transplant to those who need to and want to know. We both had the same objective: patient education in the form of a book to be used as a resource for information on solid organ transplantation. However, we approached the goal from two distinctive perspectives. My impression of what it would take to accomplish this huge task was simple. . . . Write down everything I know about solid organ transplant! I had been a nurse for over twenty years and had worked in transplant in some capacity for ten. My part, I thought, was easy, I have since realized my naivete. When I am face to face with a potential transplant recipient, a confused family, a newly transplanted patient, or for that matter, my peers and multidisciplinary team, I can easily sense their concern, acknowledge their understanding, or simply recognize the fact that I need to repeat myself, rephrase my response, or even gesture with my hands to get my point across. Not so with the written word. For this book I have agonized over my explanations, amended my original thoughts, and expanded on written words in an attempt to get my point across clearly and concisely so that transplant is a more understandable process for those who care to learn.

Elizabeth's vast knowledge of the English language, and her experience as a recipient of a liver transplant, is what has really made this book available to you today. She knew what it would take to accomplish this task and set forth to do it. She is the substance placed on these pages; I just set her straight on the facts!

—Janet B. Mize, RN, BSN, CCTC, CMC

Being told that you may need an organ transplant may be the most frightening news you will ever receive. It was for me. Of course, having been diagnosed with end-stage liver disease, I had no other option. I searched for information on transplantation upon receiving my diagnosis in 1993, so that I could learn about what I was in for and ease my anxiety. As I had been a teacher for most of my life, I immediately looked for a textbook. Where was it? Surely in some medical library, at a university, at a city library, at a bookstore. Guess again. There was plenty of information available for clinical practitioners, which was often written by physicians for physicians. Yet, with the exception of a few monographs from the American Liver Foundation, there was nothing available for the layperson.

I would come to learn that a member of the transplant team—the nurse coordinator—was my most precious source of information. My textbook was in the coordinator's head, but she carried that around exclusively. The education available at once-a-month support group meetings gradually acquainted me with the mysterious world of transplantation. I remain most grateful for that information, but I also remember how difficult it was not to be able to take it home. I couldn't hand it to a loved one who was as racked as I was by the diagnosis. At the same time, I felt it was my place—because it was my illness—to reassure my family and friends.

This is the book I didn't have and that I so desperately wanted. It is the material that walked around in my nurse coordinator's head, for she is the one and same Janet Mize who is my coauthor (or I am hers). Sometimes her knowledge is expressed in this book through my voice, sometimes in her own words. Together we will offer the information you need—the basic facts and advice, as well as some issues you may not have been aware of.

I hope you can benefit from my personal experience with transplantation. I was able to return to teaching ten months after transplant; I have lived a full and satisfying life since then. With a book like this in mind, I worked toward and received a doctorate in the medical humanities focusing much of the course work and my dissertation on coping with transplantation.

Janet Mize coordinates organ transplants, which means that, among other things, she educates recipients about expectations, techniques, and protocols pertaining to transplantation. She sees her patients through the long ordeal and counsels them along the way. Janet is now the transplant administrator at the University of California, Irvine. She also knows firsthand about the anxiety of the transplant patient's family—her husband, David, is a liver recipient.

In this book Janet and I take you through every step of your journey, from organ candidacy to long-term transplantation recovery. It is our hope that this book will serve you as a close companion during your journey toward better health.

—Elizabeth Parr, Ph.D.

Introduction

If you selected this book, it is likely that you already know that you are in a waiting line for an organ transplant, or perhaps you have a loved one who is. You have been confronted with an awesome, terrifying situation about which you, like most of the population, know little or nothing. You have a million questions concerning transplantation. You worry about survival rate, the actual procedure, and the impact of this radical alteration on your family. Perhaps you know a little bit about the medical successes—more and more people are having transplants and are returning to normal lives afterward. What you don't know, however, is *how* they survived and *how* they coped, psychologically or emotionally.

This book is full of answers to your questions, even those that are as yet unconscious, unspoken. You will read about the facts of transplantation, the meanings of medical terms, the purposes of medications, and techniques and strategies for coping and for healing. The first part of the book discusses the experience of the organ transplant candidate, as he or she waits for an organ that meets the necessary specifications. This initial phase may be the most challenging. You will need strategies for keeping your spirits up; so much depends on your physical and emotional well-being as you approach the transplant surgery. The second part addresses the surgery itself, so that you will have a clear idea of what occurs in the operating room and, afterward, in the intensive care unit. The third part of this book introduces you to life after transplant, with further suggestions for taking care of the new organ and for coping with your new lifestyle.

There is no doubt that you are a unique person, and you will be a unique organ recipient. You bring a lifetime of personal coping skills to this new adventure. This book will help you learn to place those skills and others in this new context of surviving organ transplantation. The book has been written to calm your fears and prepare you mentally and emotionally for each step of the procedure. We know that we can help; we have been where you are.

Remember that knowledge is power; and the more you feel your own power, the better you will cope. We are dedicated to the idea that the more you understand the illness and the transplantation process, the more you will be able to participate in your own healing or the healing of your loved one. After transplant, your involvement becomes even more important, because you will be more or less on your own. The preservation of that valuable new organ is truly up to the recipient. So, are you ready for an education you never dreamed of undertaking? Let's go.

PART ONE

Pre-Transplant

CHAPTER ONE

Common Solid Organ Transplants

As of October 2000, more than 77,000 people were registered on the UNOS (United Network for Organ Sharing) waiting list. Of these, about 66 percent were awaiting kidney transplantation, and 17 percent were awaiting liver transplantation. The remaining 17 percent awaited hearts, lungs, and pancreases. There are more than twenty thousand transplants performed each year. On the average, eleven to twelve patients die each day while awaiting a transplant. These are sobering statistics. From what causes did so many people become so very ill?

A solid organ transplant is the removal of a defective liver, kidney, pancreas, heart, lung, or other major organ and replacing it with another from a donor's body. Why would a person have to undergo the radical therapy of organ transplant? What has happened to our own organs that we must give them up and replace them with another's? This chapter addresses how you and I got here—how we arrived at the end stage of an organ disease—through a discussion of the various kinds of solid organ transplants, describing what circumstances might necessitate each type.

The Heart

The heart is a muscular organ that lies near the center of the chest. Its primary function is to supply the body with oxygen while ridding it of carbon dioxide. It pumps the body's oxygen-depleted blood into the lungs, which remove the carbon dioxide from the blood and replenish its oxygen. The heart then pumps the reoxygenated blood back to the tissues of the body. When things go wrong with the heart, it is a serious situation.

In the United States, cardiovascular diseases claim eight hundred thousand lives annually. Those cardiovascular disorders that lead to heart failure are generally those that precipitate the need for a heart transplant. Heart failure is a condition in which the heart is unable to pump enough blood to meet the body's needs for everyday functions.

Heart failure is characterized by shortness of breath, especially when one lies down at night. The patient complains of fatigue and poor exercise tolerance. He or she cannot climb a flight of stairs or walk a block without some chest discomfort, shortness of breath, and/or chest pain. Sometimes these symptoms are accompanied by congestion in the lungs and edema (swelling due to fluid retention) in the extremities.

Generally, doctors attempt to treat heart failure with medication, corrective surgery, or treatment of the underlying cause (obesity, smoking, poor diet, etc.). If treatment does not work, heart transplantation is considered for otherwise healthy patients.

The two most common causes of heart failure that result in the need for transplantation are cardiomyopathy and coronary artery disease. Cardiomyopathy is a disease of the heart muscle that reduces the strength of the heart's contractions and hence decreases the efficiency of blood circulation. Symptoms might include fatigue, chest pain, and palpitations. Coronary artery disease is a disease of the blood vessel that carries blood away from the left ventricle (lower chamber) of the heart through the aorta (the largest artery in the body) to other parts of the body. Two manifestations of this disease are chest pain, also known as angina, usually associated with effort or anxiety, and heart attack.

Selection of adult heart transplant recipient is based upon the clinical determination of which patients are most likely to exhibit substantial improvement in functional capacity and in life expectancy. Earlier patient-selection guidelines have been broadened over the past two decades and are based on those preoperative characteristics associated with the best patient survival and greatest degree of rehabilitation following surgery. Symptoms that are not controllable with medications and poor one-year prognosis with conventional medical or surgical treatment are common characteristics of all patients considered for transplantation.

Those patients on continuous-medication support or those on a mechanical-assist device are most likely to remain hospitalized and receive a priority on the waiting list. Those patients with moderate heart failure symptoms stabilized with the use of oral medications and awaiting a heart at home run a much higher risk of suffering a fatal event during their wait. Most patients are treated conservatively with medical management. It is important to remember that all options should be exhausted before transplant is considered.

The Lungs

The lungs are the largest part of the respiratory system. Their functions are to remove carbon dioxide (the waste product of respiration) from oxygen-depleted blood, which is pumped into the lungs by the heart, and then to oxygenate the blood, which the heart then pumps back to the body's tissues.

Because the heart and lungs work so closely together, often problems with the lungs cause eventual heart problems. Chronic pulmonary diseases cause difficulty in getting blood flow to the right side of the heart. In these situations, there are two organs failing, and so the patient may need both organs transplanted. Depending on the extent of damage, one may need a single lung transplant, a double-lung transplant, or a heart-lung transplant.

Signs of lung problems (respiratory failure) include breathing difficulties; cyanosis (bluish discoloration of the skin); chest pain; wheezing or crowing sound produced in the chest upon breathing; confusion; sleepiness—even loss of consciousness; deep, rapid breathing; and coma.

There are no universal agreed-upon standards for listing for lung transplant. Patients whose pulmonary function and prognosis justify transplantation and whose current health will not increase the risk of the operation unnecessarily or jeopardize its long-term success are considered for transplant.

The Kidneys

The kidneys are bean-shaped organs located on either side of the middle abdomen. The primary functions of the kidneys are to filter waste and excessive sodium and water from the body and to help eliminate them from the body as urine. If the kidneys are not functioning properly—kidney failure, also called renal failure—metabolic waste products build up in the blood, in effect poisoning the body. Signs of kidney failure include frequent urination, high blood pressure, fatigue, muscle weakness and cramps, loss of appetite, nausea and vomiting, intestinal ulcers, and severe itching. There are two types of kidney failure—acute and chronic.

Acute kidney failure is a rapid decline in kidney function. It can occur as a result of any condition that (1) decreases blood flow to the kidneys, including heart failure, liver failure, extremely low blood pressure, blood loss, blocked blood vessels, and so on; (2) obstructs the flow of urine from the kidneys; or (3) injures the kidneys, including the ingestion of toxic substances—even certain medications over long periods of time, the presence of crystals or proteins in the kidneys, and direct injury to the kidneys. Generally, acute kidney failure can be treated successfully without the need for transplantation; however, if kidney failure is severe, dialysis (see page 7) or even transplantation may be necessary.

Chronic kidney failure is slowly progressive decline in kidney function over time. It can be caused by high blood pressure; obstruction of the urinary tract; inflammation of the filtering units within the kidneys; kidney disorders, including polycystic kidney disease; diabetes mellitus; and such autoimmune disorders as lupus.

As mentioned at the beginning of this chapter, 66 percent of all registered patients for transplant on the UNOS waiting list are in need of a kidney. That is an intimidating statistic. A person's chances of receiving a kidney are about fourty thousand to one in the United States. Receiving a kidney must feel to the recipient a little like winning the lottery. Fortunately, though, if you are waiting, the selection process is not quite as random as the lottery. Indeed, you will learn that the UNOS is your friend! Its regulations sometimes chafe an enthusiastic transplant team, but the rules prevent anarchy and are meant to prevent unfair privilege in this delicately balanced field of transplantation.

DIALYSIS

Before kidney transplant is undergone, a technique for removing waste products and excess water from the blood called dialysis is often first used in kidney patients. There are two types of dialysis: hemodialysis and peritoneal dialysis.

In hemodialysis the patient's blood is pumped from the body and passed through an artificial kidney machine, which filters the toxins from the blood. The machine then returns the purified blood to the patient.

Peritoneal dialysis makes use of the body's own system. A catheter is inserted into the two-layered semipermeable membrane that lines the wall of the abdominal cavity—the peritoneum. The peritoneum works as a natural filter. A sterile fluid is pumped into the abdominal cavity. The peritoneum allows the toxic substances, but not the blood, to be filtered out.

Dialysis does the job that the failed kidneys could not of removing wastes from the blood and excess fluid from the body and restoring important elements to the body system. However, long-term dialysis can be rather inconvenient, as it requires hours-long sessions several times a week. Also, as with any invasive procedure, there is risk of infection. Often when long-term dialysis is required, the patient is ultimately placed on the waiting list for a kidney transplant after being declared by a kidney specialist, called a nephrologist, as being in end-stage renal failure.

Special tests alert the nephrologist to the patient's condition, but there are signs and symptoms such as hypertension (high blood pressure), anemia, anorexia, pericarditis (inflammation of the membrane that encloses the heart), shortness of breath, and pulmonary edema, all of which point to end-stage renal disease. If your kidney disease has progressed to end stage, and for some reason dialysis is not working for you, then you, your nephrologist, and your family may opt for organ transplantation.

Ten thousand kidney transplants are performed annually in the United States. You have probably heard heartwarming stories on television news or talk shows about the family member who heroically sacrifices a kidney so that a dear relative may live. Indeed, this is the best scenario for the kidney recipient because a tissue match is necessary for donor–recipient compatibility. Close relatives often have closely matching human leukocyte antigens (HLAs). These are white blood cells, on the surface of a person's cells, that attack foreign proteins. They act as a kind of barrier, like a reef or a fortress against harmful invaders. This close but not perfect match minimizes the chances of rejection of the donor organan. The recipient's body is more likely to "mistake" the new kidney for one of its own and hence not set its immune system against it. This is helped along, of course, by antirejection drugs.

LIVE DONOR TRANSPLANT

Sometimes the living donor to the patient in renal failure is not a blood relative but the patient's spouse. It is hard for most of us to think of this very significant other as being "unrelated," but of course, as far as tissue compatibility is concerned, though the spouse may prove to be a match, he or she is not related. While there is no clear biological advantage in these cases over other living donors, there are certainly emotional advantages. The operation can be planned; there is no stressful waiting period. There is a window of opportunity to perform the transplant when the patient is in an optimal medical condition.

Janet says: "I like the odds of live donor transplants. The recipient is often more motivated to remain compliant when the donor lives in the same house. The donor shares an interest in the medication regime, as well as being a constant reminder of that special gift."

Living-related and even nonrelated donors are a partial answer to the shortage of cadaveric kidney donors. With laparoscopic surgery, a donor may have to stay only twenty-four to forty-eight hours in the hospital. The remaining kidney enlarges eventually to take over full function. The longer a patient is on dialysis, the more susceptible he or she is to infection, to anemia, and to hyper- or hypotension (high or low blood pressure). The diabetic patient especially benefits from a living donor because his or her condition deteriorates much more quickly on dialysis than that of a non-diabetic.

The Liver

The liver is a large, complex organ. Many of its functions still are not known. It plays an important role in the metabolism of proteins, fats, carbohydrates, vitamins, and minerals; it produces half of the body's cholesterol (the rest is obtained in the diet); it produces the blood's clotting factors; and it breaks down harmful substances created in the body or absorbed from the intestine. Certainly, when the liver is not functioning properly, the body is in big trouble.

Signs of liver disease include jaundice (yellowing of the skin); portal hypertension, leading to the formation of varices (engorged veins) in the esophagus that may bleed, an enlarged spleen, and fluid in the abdomen (ascites); encephalopathy (deterioration of mental function due to buildup of toxins in the blood), which can ultimately lead to coma; fatigue; weakness; nausea; and loss of appetite. When patients have frequent bleeds, the transplant team may choose to reduce the pressure within the vessels by shunting the blood away from the liver. One popular method is called a transjugular intrahepatic portal systemic shunt (TIPSS).

Fulminant liver failure is the sudden onset of severe liver disease in a previously healthy person. It may be caused by many toxins, acute viral hepatitis, mushroom poisonings, accidental overdoses, or cumulative use of prescription drugs. Some of the sickest patients, Janet says, that she has seen were simply trying to control the pain from a common toothache and ingested too many analgesics in too short a time frame. Those who have acute onset are sicker than those who have a progression into chronic end-stage liver disease, such as that which occurs with hepatitis. These unsuspecting candidates do well following transplant, however, because there is no chronic disease process working on the otherwise healthy body.

Unfortunately, liver transplant is the only option for those with end-stage liver disease. There are currently no mechanical organ replacement devices like dialysis for the liver approved for use by the Food and Drug Administration (FDA) in the United States. Fortunately, liver transplant is the most effective (and the most expensive) of all transplant procedures. If successful, liver transplant can bring the fastest and greatest improvements in the quality of life of the recipient. A few investigational devices are being tested for their effectiveness in treating liver failure due to toxins and prove to be promising in the near future. At the present time, liver transplant is the most effective means of saving life but does not come without costs. Liver transplantation is one of the most difficult and pricey surgeries available today. When successful, liver transplant is the better treatment option to improve the quality of life of the patient suffering from end-stage liver disease. The following conditions can necessitate liver transplantation.

CIRRHOSIS

Cirrhosis is the formation of nonfunctioning scar tissue, destroying normal liver tissue. In the United States, about one in seventy people dies as the direct result of chronic liver disease and cirrhosis. Heavy alcohol consumption, the use of certain drugs and exposure to certain chemicals, infection (hepatitis), autoimmune disorders such as lupus, diabetes, accumulation of too much iron and copper in the liver, and obstruction of the liver's bile ducts are among the causes of cirrhosis.

PRIMARY BILIARY CIRRHOSIS

Primary biliary cirrhosis is inflammation of the bile ducts—the vessels through which bile exits the liver. Bile is a liquid produced by the liver that aids in digestion. This inflammation leads to scarring and blockage of the bile duct. Scarring eventually spreads to the entire liver. Biliary atresia, a congenital condition in which the infant's bile ducts developed either abnormally or not at all, can lead to biliary cirrhosis if left untreated.

HEPATITIS

Hepatitis is inflammation of the liver, which can lead to cell damage. It is most often caused by a virus, most commonly one of six hepatitis viruses: A, B, C, D, E, or G. Transmission of hepatitis A is usually the result of poor hygiene, as the virus is primarily found in the stool of an infected person.

Hepatitis B is present in the blood and other body fluids of infected people. It is spread sexually and through blood contact by such means as needle sharing, razor sharing, ear piercing, and tattooing. Many cases of hepatitis B were contracted from the use of infected blood transfused prior to strict regulatory interventions in the early 1980s. In certain cases the virus may lead to chronic hepatitis and eventually to liver cirrhosis and/or liver cancer.

Hepatitis C is the cause of most transfusion-associated hepatitis cases. These are those cases in which the patient received blood transfusion before 1992, the date after which blood and blood products were carefully screened for the virus previously known as Type non-A/non-B. It may remain in the system of the infected person for many years before manifesting. About 5 percent of hepatitis C–infected people will progress to cirrhosis, often as long as twenty years after infection. Hepatitis C is mainly a blood-borne disease. There are approximately 110,000 persons in the United States today with hepatitis C. Not all of these will progress to liver transplant.

Hepatitis can also be caused by excessive consumption of alcohol or certain drugs. In autoimmune hepatitis, the body's immune system attacks its own liver, leading to liver damage. Hepatitis can be either acute or chronic.

Acute hepatitis is that which lasts fewer than six months. It is rarely so serious that it causes liver failure; though infection with the hepatitis B virus is generally acute *and* can be very serious and even fatal. Chronic hepatitis develops over years.

PRIMARY LIVER TUMORS

Those with liver cancer may be considered candidates for liver transplantation only if the tumors are confined to the liver. Unfortunately, liver cancer often is not detected until it has been present for some time and has had time to spread.

METABOLIC LIVER DISORDERS

There are also disorders of metabolism that can lead to liver disease and failure. Hemochromatosis is a genetic condition that causes the body to absorb and store too much iron. While iron is an essential mineral for good health, too much of it is toxic to the body. Fortunately, this disorder is easily treatable when detected early; however, left untreated, it can lead to cirrhosis and liver failure. Relatives of patients identified with hemachromatosis should be tested for the disease by a simple blood test.

Wilson's disease is an inherited disorder in which the liver does not secrete copper, another essential mineral that is toxic in large amounts, into the bloodstream. As a result, copper accumulates in the liver and nervous system, leading to severe liver and neurological disease. Liver transplantation is indicated for those with very advanced disease. Following transplant, these patients recover, often reversing all neurological problems.

ALCOHOLIC LIVER DISEASE

Alcoholic liver disease (ALD), or alcoholic cirrhosis, is liver damage caused by excessive, prolonged consumption of alcohol. The single most important criterion for the patient with ALD is the absolute abstinence from alcohol and the declared understanding that this is a permanent lifestyle modification. Once the patient stops drinking, progression of scarring and damage ceases, although liver damage is irreversible.

If damage is so severe that a transplant is necessary for survival, the patient will not even be considered for transplant unless he or she has stopped drinking and has been evaluated extensively and has been deemed to have a reduced risk of returning to drinking. Each transplant center has its own regulations, but on average they require six months to one year of sobriety with documentation of attendance at Alcoholics Anonymous. Attendance at Narcotics Anonymous is mandated for those who have damaged their liver by illicit drug use. The patient, upon being listed for transplant, often is asked to sign a contract stating that he or she will not drink or use drugs and will submit to random drug screening while awaiting transplantation.

The Pancreas

The pancreas is a glandular organ, about five inches long, that is considered to be part of both the digestive and the endocrine systems. It consists of two basic types of tissue: the acini, which produce digestive enzymes, and the islets, which produce hormones that control blood-sugar levels—insulin and glucagon. While dysfunction can certainly occur in the digestive-system portion of the pancreas, pancreas transplant is performed only for problems with the secretion of insulin (a blood sugar–lowering hormone)—that is, with diabetes.

Pancreas transplantation differs from most other transplants in that it is usually not done as a last-resort, life-saving measure but rather is performed on those with Type I diabetes (where the pancreas ceases producing insulin), to prevent some of the life-threatening complications that can occur with diabetes, and on those whose insulin levels are not well controlled with insulin injections.

Trauma or Crohn's disease, a chronic inflammatory gastrointestinal disease that can affect any part of the gastrointestinal tract, can also necessitate transplant.

In addition to transplantation of the whole pancreas, transplantation of the islet cells can also be performed. This is a relatively new and experimental procedure, but results thus far appear promising.

A combined kidney-pancreas transplant is usually performed on diabetes mellitus Type I patients with end-stage renal failure. Diabetes can be the cause of renal failure in 40 percent of patients requiring dialysis.

One of the controversies in medical circles surrounding pancreas or islet cell transplants is the issue of immunosuppressant drugs. As you will learn later in this book, the immune systems of transplant recipients must be suppressed so their bodies do not try to reject their new organ or organs. In cases where transplant is essential for life, this situation is inevitable, but with pancreas transplant, the question is whether long-term complications of diabetes mellitus are more or less significant than the possible long-term complications of immunosuppression. You will read about the effects of immunosuppressant antirejection drugs on the transplant recipient in Parts Two and Three.

The Small Intestine

After food is swallowed it goes from the stomach, where it begins to be broken down, to the small intestine, where it is further digested and its nutrients are absorbed into the bloodstream. Transplant is considered when the small intestine is unable to absorb nutrients. Because the gut will not absorb nutrients needed for metabolism, nutrients must be supplied to the patient by intravenous (IV) therapy. The condition is often seen in pediatric patients as a congenital abnormality, and the transplant is sometimes done with a liver transplant: liver–small bowel. Another common reason for this procedure is surgical, that is, when the patient loses the small bowel to resection (usually in surgery for a nonmalignant tumor or polyp) or a blockage or some trauma has left a patient without enough healthy bowel to absorb nutrients.

Conclusion

Whew! This lesson in biology is over. Perhaps it was more than you ever wanted to know about your body and its vulnerability to damage. A virus, our family genes, trauma like that which occurs in an automobile accident, or, sadly, our own abuse of our bodies can make us so ill that an organ transplant is our only recourse if we want to return to good health.

So, now that you've been diagnosed, and your family doctor has offered a prognosis and course of treatment, where do you go from here? Read on!

CHAPTER TWO

Determining Candidacy for Transplantation

If Janet were able to have a conversation with you, she would tell you, as she told me, that upon learning from your physician that you need an organ transplant, it is up to you to investigate your options. Let that be the first thing you learn about transplant. *You* make the decisions; you and only you can decide if transplant is the option for you. In the case of transplantation of the life-saving organs—liver, heart, and lungs—it may be the decision whether you live or die. In the case of kidney or kidney-pancreas transplantation, you are looking at alternatives to improve your lifestyle. If dialysis or daily injections of insulin limit you or cause undue side effects, then maybe transplant is an appropriate alternative treatment to your disease management. Transplant, however, may not always be a life-saving procedure. There are risks associated with transplant and with living in an immune-suppressed state. These risks need to be weighed when making your decision.

The road to recovery is not always an easy one, and your choice will certainly have an impact on your family. Explore each option carefully; make the best decision you can; and don't look back. It is important to go down your chosen path equipped with the knowledge and determination to do whatever it takes to make it work, knowing that there may be stumbling blocks along the way.

Determining transplantation candidacy begins with a period in which the potential transplant candidate is evaluated. This evaluation includes a series of rigorous tests. The results of these tests indicate whether or not an organ transplant is the right course for the particular patient; and if the answer is yes, the patient becomes a transplant candidate.

This chapter gives information about the testing process, about certain indications that transplant is not in order for a person, and about organ donation and distribution in the United States. We begin with my story as a kind of prototype. It is not unlike some of your stories, I'm sure.

Elizabeth's Road Toward Candidacy

It was a March day in 1992. It was not springlike yet. I believe that it was an early Saturday evening, and I was propped comfortably on a couch, grading papers. I suddenly felt severely nauseated and headed for the bathroom. I don't remember feeling ill beforehand. To my shock and horror, I vomited blood—a lot of it. Initially, I took no action while I tried to sort things out. Ultimately, I called a friend who took me to the emergency room.

I was seen in the emergency room by a surgeon who told me that I had a bleeding stomach ulcer and that my liver enzyme activity was elevated. The bleeding had stopped, however. I was hospitalized for observation for two or three days. After discharge, I went about my business, though I was more careful about nutrition and abstaining from alcohol and any other provoking substance.

Almost one year later, I experienced another "bleed," as the doctors called it. I returned to the emergency room, only this time I was unconscious; in fact I was comatose. The voices around and above me did not think that I would wake up. They suggested life support. To their surprise, I awoke twenty-four hours later sane, very weak, even more afraid than the first time, and feeling helpless, not knowing what to do.

For the year that passed between bleeds, I had regularly visited the internist who treated me at the hospital when my "ulcer" had been diagnosed. After my first emergency room visit, I had been referred to a gastroenterologist who, observing my blood tests, knew that I had a serious liver disease

and mentioned that, down the line, I might require a transplant. (When my
mother was pregnant with one of my brothers, her condition had been initially diagnosed as a gallbladder problem by a wonderful, reputable gyne-
cologist. Some of my mother's friends told the doctor, upon meeting him one
day in the hospital elevator, that they were on the way to the nursery to "see
Elizabeth's gallbladder." Physicians really don't know everything.) This
doctor was really rather casual about the whole thing, and I was sure that it
would never come to that. Of course it wouldn't. Somehow or other, I wouldn't
allow it. I was sure that a transplant meant that I would die on the table.

All I knew about transplants was about that doctor in South Africa in
the 1960s who had performed a heart transplant on some poor soul who
lived only a few days. Even my experience in 1992 happened before all
the public service announcements and current news broadcasts about
transplantation. The public was not informed about the progress being
made in organ donation and transplantation, and I guess I just wasn't interested. Well, *this* got my attention.

After the second bleed, I began looking for help with a trusty friend at
my side. Ordinarily, a patient is referred by his or her family physician or
primary care physician (PCP) to a specialist, who may then in turn refer
the patient to a transplant center—or the PCP may refer the patient directly to a transplant center nearby. This, however, is not always the case.
Many times potential transplantees must do their own legwork or surf the
Internet, because some practicing physicians have not studied the still-
emerging field of transplantation and simply do not think of it as a possible medical treatment. In my case, I had to find a center that I found
viable. After having located the center, about a mile from my home, I did
the honorable and the valiant thing—I had my friend call the transplant
coordinator (who turned out to be Janet), pretend that she was me, get information, and make an appointment. I remember the clinic visit that followed vividly, as I am sure you will (or do).

After a time in the waiting room, I was called to go down a hall (which
seemed at least fifty miles long) at the end of which I visualized an elec-
tric chair. I had my friend accompany me. We sat in a small examining
room. You know the kind—instruments of torture within easy reach, space
about four feet by four feet—a cell, in other words.

In came Janet, full of enthusiasm and kindness. I cried then, probably for the first time that day. That cry was succeeded by others on that day and the following days—one for each medical visitor: the specialist and the surgeon, and ultimately the social worker, the psychiatrist, and the medical ethicist. My initial visits to medical specialists were the first opportunities for me to be able to say out loud that I had a really serious liver disease—that I was afraid that I might die. I hadn't heard the comforting term *end-stage* yet. That term would eventually get thrown around and would "cheer me up" even further.

Whereas before I had refused to think about transplant as an option, now I could think of no other. So I initiated a long effort of determination, which would see me through months of complicated tests, additional sickness and treatments, and too much waiting.

We have already mentioned the stress of waiting for the transplant candidate. That period can stretch into months. It can be complicated, in the case of heart and kidney and lung transplants, by the need to rely on assist devices—mechanical organs. We discuss at length some coping techniques for this long, empty-feeling pretransplant period later. First let's get you through the earliest period of candidacy and the procedures involved.

The Process

When I first learned that I needed an organ transplant, I didn't know what to expect. I also didn't realize how long and complicated the process of determining my candidacy for transplant would be. My doctor had determined that I needed a transplant. Wasn't that enough? I would quickly learn that it was not. The following are steps that must be taken in determining your candidacy for transplant.

FINDING A CENTER

Once a doctor determines that a patient requires an organ transplant, the doctor will refer the patient to his or her center of choice, which is usually local if possible. Sometimes the doctor refers a patient to a transplant center covered by the patient's insurance. In many cases, the patient may have to travel some distance just to have insurance coverage.

A helpful resource may be the National Transplant Assistance Fund (NTAF), a not-for-profit resource association for transplant patients, their families, and those who service them. The Fund can provide you with a list of transplant centers and information on centers appropriate for your specific requirements. According to the NTAF, several insurance companies often negotiate price discounts with certain transplant centers, thus covering transplantation only for patients who undergo the procedure at their contracted center. Patients can be forced to move hundreds of miles to be treated at the center their insurance designates, even though there may be an equally qualified center closer to home. Be aware that when the patient chooses to remain in his or her own community at a noncontracted center, coverage may be denied and the entire cost of transplantation may need to be raised. The NTAF may be reached at (800) 642-8399.

In selecting a center, among the first questions you should ask are "What is the total number of transplants performed at this center?" and "What are the survival rates at this center?" There are also questions you should ask of yourself: How does the location of the hospital suit you, especially with regard to your support system in that area (family, friends)? What is your general feeling about the hospital and its transplant team? Rapport will be extremely important as you progress through transplantation.

When you visit the center for your testing and evaluation, you will be interviewed by some members of the transplant team. It may not seem like an interview, but it is.

INTERVIEWS FOR TRANSPLANT CANDIDACY

The most important thing to remember when talking with any member of the transplant team is to sell yourself to them. They see many potential candidates every day. You must let them know why it is important that you receive a transplant and that you are committed to that decision. Those potential candidates who display the motivation to pursue transplant are the ones who see it through. It is important to the transplant team that they sell themselves to you as well. As transplant centers pop up across the United

States, customer satisfaction, quality care, and good outcomes are important as selling points to the center.

The beginning of the screening interview is much like a typical visit to a physician for an annual checkup. Your vital signs will be checked—especially your body temperature, because a fever usually indicates infection: a contraindication for transplant. You will be weighed and measured, have your blood drawn, and be sent home with a quart (!) container for deposit of urine over a twenty-four-hour period. Sometimes a stool sample is also required at this time. You will also be asked a million questions (most of which you have already answered) regarding your medical history and current condition.

. . . With the Transplant Coordinator

After the testing, you will meet with the transplant coordinator. I was first interviewed by Janet, the transplant team's nurse coordinator. We met in one of several examining rooms in the area of the university hospital dedicated to gastroenterology. Larger centers will have an area dedicated exclusively to transplantation. Janet began by taking a general medical history, including what was known about my family medical history. The close friend who was to become my primary caregiver was present at all of the interviews. Not only is a spouse, relative, or friend allowed to be present, they are encouraged. A caregiver is essential throughout the transplant process. In fact, the absence of one may be a negative factor that may persuade the team against transplant.

Janet gave me an overview of what I might expect in the future during the interview process. Shortly after this initial interview, she gave me a printed schedule of the times and places of testings.

. . . With the Transplant Physician

The meeting with the transplant physician, in my case a hepatologist, also began with a medical history, but she focused on those experiences that may have caused my liver disease. It makes sense, of course, that the specialist will be the first to ask about the origin and course of a specific disease. It had already been determined that I had cirrhosis of the liver, so she asked about such habits as drinking, smoking, and the use of recreational drugs. She asked whether I had ever had hepatitis, and in regard to that, where I had traveled. She asked if I had ever gotten a tattoo or ear piercing. In other words, the physician interview will be disease specific.

. . . With the Transplant Surgeon

In some centers it may be a while before the patient meets a surgeon. In my case, I was interviewed by one of the transplant surgeons early, before testing began. Again, he was specialty specific and asked, among other questions, whether I had ever had surgery. He was pleased to learn that I had no surgical scars. Internal surgical scar tissue can cause adhesions (tissue that "sticks together"), complicating transplantation. I did not meet with the chief transplant surgeon until after I had undergone many tests and the committee had decided to accept me as a candidate.

Other Interviews

Before being accepted for transplant candidacy, a potential candidate may have to meet with several other members of a transplant-candidacy committee. The patient will be interviewed by a staff psychologist or psychiatrist. This mental health professional will be available to assist the candidate/recipient and the team throughout the transplant process. In the initial interview, he or she will also assess the patient's potential for successful transplant. The psychologist or psychiatrist will ask questions that will help determine the potential candidate's abilities to cope with a transplant, the lifestyle changes it will bring, and the nature of his or her support system. In addition, you might meet with a nutritionist, a financial advisor, and a social worker.

TESTING

Janet's view of the evaluation process is that it is much like a "honeymoon period" for you and the transplant team. Relationships are made and trust is built between the patient and his or her family and the transplant team. The testing required prior to candidate selection is not only used to evaluate a patient's overall health but it also tells the transplant team how dependable you are. In a way, the purpose of the evaluation is not only to rule out any medical or technical reason that you should not undergo transplant, but also to see what you do with direction, because much of your pre- and post-transplant period will consist of just that—following direction. A transplant candidate who does not show up for scheduled appointments, does not call to reschedule missed appointments, or does not follow the instructions given to him or her by the transplant coordinator may be perceived by the team as not being dependable.

Likewise, you must be sure that you find the team dependable. An evaluation should take into consideration the patient's condition; dialysis schedule, if applicable; transportation needs; and other specific needs, including those regarding mobility and dietary restrictions. Schedules that ignore these considerations tell the patient something about the team. This is a team effort, and you are an important member of the team, whose only focus should be to get you through transplantation successfully.

Prior tests from a primary care physician or specialist are usually accepted, and the patient need not repeat them in the candidacy determination process if they were recently conducted. Required tests are similar for all solid organ candidates. A doctor may choose to run other tests, but candidates may expect the following, regardless of the failing organ.

A thorough heart evaluation is done. Depending on age, a stress test recording the motion and regularity of the heart muscle during exercise may be needed. If your condition does not permit actual exercise on a treadmill, there are medications that can be given that evoke an exercise response. A heart tracing to access your heart rate and rhythm will also be done. All of these results will be reviewed by a cardiologist who predicts your heart's ability to accept the rigors of a major surgery. The cardiologist you see works closely with the transplant team to ensure there are no complications attributed to your heart's function.

A pulmonary (lung) function evaluation is done to predict lung volumes and capacity. This is important in the immediate post-operative period when oxygenation is needed to promote healing and provide the newly transplanted organ with blood rich in oxygen. There must be no active tuberculosis or fungal infection, either of which could be fatal once the transplant recipient is immunosuppressed with anti-rejection drugs following transplant. If a history of lung disease is discovered, then a lung physician (pulmonologist) is called for a consult. The patient is evaluated and, if needed, treatments for such diseases as tuberculosis can delay transplant up to a year.

Your kidney function is evaluated. The kidneys must be healthy prior to a patient's undergoing transplant. This series of tests is significant even if the solid organ being replaced is not the kidney. These tests can include, but not be limited to, cultures of urine, twenty-four-hour urine collection for protein, and creatinine clearance. If any test is reported abnormal, a nephrologist (a kidney specialist) will be consulted to conduct further tests. A general physical exam will be performed if the patient has not had such an examination within the past year. Expect many of these physical examinations during your evaluation. Janet says to keep in mind that it is the summary of all the examinations and physician consultations that support your candidacy to transplant. The team can request a CAT scan, also known as CT scan usually focused on the body area which houses the organ in need for transplant. A series of these may be done during your evaluation. It provides a cross-sectional image of the tissue or body being examined. This special x-ray requires preparation that usually entails mixing and drinking a liquid the night before the procedure. This test also requires that you not eat or drink anything for at least six hours before your testing time. If you are a diabetic, please consult your transplant coordinator to receive specific instructions for this and any test requiring that you fast for a period of time prior to the test/procedure.

An ultrasound scan of the failing organ is always performed for liver and kidney patients. The ultrasound can help the physicians determine whether or not the veins and arteries of the organ are intact; these will be connected at surgery to the new organ. The size of the liver and kidneys informs the physician of the stage of organ deterioration. Ultrasounds allow the transplant team to rule out any masses in either organ.

Generally, patients should have a dental examination within a year of the evaluation. The routine dental examination is important to your health following transplant. All dental work that needs to be done should be done prior to transplantation, as a dental infection following transplant can lead to bacteria being spread and vegetating in and around your heart valves. This could damage the heart valves that pump the blood through the body.

This condition, known as endocarditis, could delay or even eliminate the possibility of receiving a solid organ transplant. Routine dental examinations should be scheduled while you await the transplant, because afterward, while the transplant team is working to adjust critical levels of medication and you are on larger doses of steroids and are more prone to infection (for three to six months), dental work is not recommended.

CONTRAINDICATIONS FOR TRANSPLANT

There are some problems that may cause the members of a transplant team to refuse some patients as candidates for those precious, scarce organs. These problems are called contraindications—indicators, such as other conditions present, that transplantation is inadvisable. Some of the general contraindications for solid organ transplant include:

- Advanced age or disease.
- Lack of social support or adequate support system to allow for successful rehabilitation.
- Systemic infection unresponsive to antibiotics.

Following are some additional contraindications for transplant.

Lack of Stamina

The candidate must be in sufficient physical condition to withstand the transplant procedure. This general physical wellness is determined by the tests outlined above and continuous medical monitoring during the evaluation and wait for transplant. Given the long waiting period for the availability of a suitable organ, the transplant team must ascertain the potential candidate's ability to endure the wait. Understand that those who have the luxury (relatively good health) of waiting for transplant are those who routinely have the better outcomes. Patients in urgent need are often very ill, and maintaining a status quo becomes a moot point: keeping the patient alive and free of infection to get the first available organ becomes the issue at that point. We presume here, for the sake of outlining the transplant process, that the candidate is stable and not in acute organ failure. When it is finally time for the transplant, the patient must be able to tolerate the long surgery. Surgeries for some organs last as long as sixteen hours, require multiple blood transfusions, as well as medical interventions to maintain bodily functions.

Metastasis of Cancer

To be eligible for solid organ transplant, a patient must show no signs of a cancerous tumor that has spread to another part of the body. If a primary cancer exists, it must be contained in the organ involved in transplant. There are cancers for which a primary tumor may have been removed and chemotherapy given before the patient is listed for transplant. In these situations (ovarian cancer, prostate cancer, lung cancer), patients are evaluated on an individual basis and routinely judged appropriate candidates for transplant if there is no recurrence for three to five years before being considered for transplant. Frequent examinations (x-ray and blood work) should be done to detect early signs of recurrence of cancer. The immune system of the transplant recipient, until someone invents a magic bullet, will be suppressed. The system of an immune-suppressed person cannot fight off the spread of malignancy. In ordinary circumstances, the body's immune system reacts to antigens (foreign proteins) such as cancer cells by producing antibodies to destroy them. In the immune-suppressed person, this ability is minimal or absent. In other words, the cancer can attack the new organ all over again. You will learn more about immune suppression and the drugs you will be taking to suppress your immune system after transplant in subsequent chapters.

Multisystem Organ Failure

If the patient is suffering from multisystem organ failure, so that the transplant of a single solid organ would not improve his or her overall health, then transplantation is not a viable therapy. The exception to this rule is when a second organ is failing due to the failure of a primary organ, most commonly, kidney failure as a result of worsening liver failure. Often the kidneys will recover following a successful liver transplant. In some cases, however, a liver-kidney transplant is required to improve quality of life.

Conclusion

So now you have presented yourself at the transplant center, gone through a battery of tests, been considered by a ponderous committee, and been judged to be healthy enough to withstand transplant. You are officially a candidate. It has a kind of solemn ring to it, like you are in the military or in preparation for job training or higher education. You feel like celebrating, but on your current nutrition regimen consisting of no salt, no fatty foods, no alcohol, and so on, how are you going to do that? Dig in and start getting ready for wellness, for a healthy life beyond transplant.

CHAPTER THREE

Who and What Are Involved in Preparing for Your Transplant

Have you ever owned anything that was custom-made—a suit, drapes, shoes? As a candidate for organ transplantation, you are about to enter a custom-made world. You will become the beneficiary of a custom-made medical management system. You will have an entire transplant team standing by who will prescribe and assist you with the medications and treatment that will sustain you until your transplant surgery. Actually, you will increasingly become the most important member of this team, aiding the others with your enthusiastic cooperation. This chapter looks closely at how the pre-transplantation process molds to your specific needs through a team of helpful individuals and through customized medication programs.

The Transplant Team

To be certified by the United Network for Organ Sharing (UNOS), a transplant center is required to meet certain criteria. Among these criteria, the transplant team must consist of a transplant surgeon, certified in solid organ transplantation or its equivalent, whose exclusive concern is transplantation, and a physician who is board certified in his or her field of specialization whose task is the medical management of the patient. A coordinator specialized in care of transplant recipients is required as well. The coordinator is the team member who is responsible for the daily operations of the center and is the one who has the most contact with the patients. Centers usually have a senior coordinator and subordinate, organ-specific coordinators. There may be a patient educator, someone who assists the busy coordinators with educating the potential recipient about the transplant process. There must also be a financial coordinator, dedicated to researching and advising according to each candidate's financial needs, and a social worker, who should have experience with transplant patients and is available twenty-four hours a day, as the rest of the team is. A psychiatrist is available for transplant patients and is very important for pre-transplant evaluation. Most transplant centers have a nutritionist or dietician who is available to transplant patients and recipients.

THE TRANSPLANT SURGEON

The transplant surgeon is the head of the team. He or she sees the patient during the evaluation process and perhaps once or twice before transplant and daily during your hospital stay. After discharge, the surgeon will still be in charge of your care. The transplant physicians are consulted, but the surgeon is the one who makes the decisions. He or she sees the patient during the post-transplant period of up to six months. After six months, most of the recipient's care is managed by the transplant physician, or the patient is referred back to the primary care physician, unless there are postoperative surgical complications.

THE TRANSPLANT PHYSICIAN

The physician is the medical director of the team, who works in conjunction with the surgeon on preoperative care of the patient while he or she waits for an organ. This doctor may be a nephrologist or urologist for the

kidney patient, a hepatologist for the patient with liver disease, a cardiologist for the heart patient, or a pulmonologist for the patient with lung disease.

THE TRANSPLANT COORDINATOR

Considered the liaison between the patient and other members of the team
both pre- and post-transplant, the transplant coordinator is a major source
of support for the patient and his or her family. Questions before and after
transplant are directed to the coordinator, who, in turn, advises and directs
concerns to the transplant team. The coordinator builds a relationship
with the patient during the usually long wait for an available organ. If
there is not a bond, says Janet, then the likelihood of a successful transplant is lessened, because communication is not effective. Little things
that can make or break a successful transplant get missed. Trust must be
established between patient and coordinator.

THE SOCIAL WORKER

The social worker understands the governmental systems and can help patients and families with funding sources. He or she also sees the patient
during evaluation for candidacy and, with the psychiatrist, helps determine the patient's ability to understand any alteration in lifestyle that he
or she must undertake with transplant. The social worker helps the patient
and family in asking questions of the team and examining concerns they
may have. The social worker is present, too, as a therapist to help the
patient and family handle stress and anxiety and to offer the team information regarding the patient's coping skills. The social worker may col-
laborate with a financial coordinator, usually an administrator from the
admitting/billing department at the transplant center. This official has a
good grasp of the dealings with the patient's insurance company, of any
contracting issues, or of anything of financial concern to the patient. The
patient can be given this information step by step by members of the team
in the transplant process.

THE PSYCHIATRIST OR PSYCHOLOGIST

The psychiatrist/psychologist not only is essential in the pre-transplant period in order to rule out any serious mental disturbances that might prevent the individual from becoming a transplant candidate but also is present throughout the process to support and clarify at the candidate's or the team's request. Serious depression may be a contraindication for transplant. The psychiatrist would be the team member to diagnose such a condition. Studies have found that patients with depression were significantly more likely to die while awaiting transplantation than the nondepressed patients. A study done on heart transplant candidates determined that there was a correlation between symptoms of heart failure and the measured level of depression. There is a connection between the psychological and the physical states in severely ill persons. The results of the study point to the necessity of supportive psychotherapeutic treatment during the stressful time of transplant, both before and after.

THE NUTRITIONIST

Sometimes the team includes a nutritionist or dietician, depending on the size of the transplant center. This professional works with families prior to transplant to develop and then help maintain an eating program appropriate to proper medical management. Certain foods in the diet can aid in healing, and certain foods can restrict or counteract the healing process. For example, before transplant, some patients must follow a salt-restricted diet and often must avoid protein, depending on the organ being transplanted; after transplant, protein is a very important element of the diet for healing. If a nutritionist is not immediately available at your local center, talk to your coordinator. He or she will help you obtain the services of a nutritionist.

THE PATIENT EDUCATOR

The team may also include a patient educator, a clinical nurse specialist who informs the patient of what to expect before and after transplant and instructs about medication prior to discharge. This position is a new one that has been created to relieve the busy coordinator. The patient educator might conduct workshops for patients and families during the evaluation period. The patient and family attend and then take a postworkshop test to check their knowledge. Patients may be given short refresher courses as they wait for transplant. This in-house educator becomes more focused on medication as the recipient gets closer to discharge post-transplant.

THE RECIPIENT

The organ recipient is also a member of this impressive transplant team. You effectively become a professional patient, as you must grow in knowledge about medication and your other exercises in your medical management. You have a new job now, and without your high job performance, all of the other transplant experts fail at theirs. Your health is their work product and their reward. Your gratitude is best demonstrated in your cooperation and finally in your wellness.

Organ Donors

Where do the donated organs come from? Since scientists cannot yet grow replacement organs (though we may be closer to that futuristic possibility than we know) we must rely on other sources: other people.

Unfortunately, it is true that someone has to die in order for someone else to receive an organ. We will take up this emotionally charged issue a little later. Actually, it is more accurate and more comforting to think about these as two separate events. Someone dies. Someone receives an organ.

Sometimes, as may be the case with liver and kidneys, the donors may be living related donors. Ten thousand kidney transplants are performed annually in the United States. You have probably heard heartwarming stories on television news or talk shows about the family member who heroically sacrifices a kidney so that a dear relative may live. Indeed, this is the best scenario for the kidney recipient because a tissue match is necessary for donor-recipient compatibility. Close relatives often have closely matching human leukocyte antigens (HLA). These are white cells that attack foreign proteins. They are present on the surface of a person's cells, and act as a kind of barrier, like a reef or a fortress against harmful invaders. They are not as likely to attack relatives. The closer the tissue match, the greater chance there will be that that transplanted organ will do well and have a long life. This close but not perfect match minimizes the chances of rejection of the donor organ. The recipient's body is more likely to "mistake" the new kidney as one of its own and hence not set its immune system against it! This is helped along, of course, by antirejection drugs. Tissue matching (HLA matching) is an important part of the decision to accept an organ for transplant for kidney and pancreas. The heart, lungs, and liver do not depend on tissue matching, but rather on size and blood type when these organs are being considered. Sometimes the living donor to the patient in renal failure is not a blood relative but the patient's spouse. It is hard for most of us to think of this very significant other as being "unrelated," but, of course, as far as tissue compatibility is concerned, though the spouse may prove to be a match he or she is not related. While there is no clear biological advantage in living donor cases, there are certainly emotional advantages. The operation can be planned; there is no stressful waiting period. There is a window of opportunity to perform the transplant when the patient is in an optimal medical condition. If you are thinking about living donor transplant, you should check with your transplant center for specific information.

Living related and even non-related donors as mentioned above are a partial answer to the shortage of cadaveric kidney donors. With laparoscopic surgery (removing the donor kidney utilizing closed circuit camera equipment through a much smaller incision), a donor may remain only 24 to 48 hours in the hospital. The remaining kidney enlarges eventually to take over full function. The longer a patient is on dialysis, the more susceptible he or she is to infection, to anemia, and hyper- or hypotension (high or low blood pressure). The diabetic patient especially benefits from a living donor kidney transplant because his condition deteriorates much more quickly on dialysis than a non-diabetic. Sometimes, as may be the case with liver and kidneys, the donors may be living related donors. Use of live donation for liver is still relatively new. This cutting-edge technology is a result of the transplants team's effort to increase the organ donor pool, eliminating the need for a long wait for a cadaveric organ and was originally developed as a mechanism to allow for more pediatric transplants. Sometimes a donated liver can be split and given to two recipients. Amazingly, a section of liver, once transplanted, will enlarge to fill the cavity. This procedure is sometimes done with two adult recipients; however, it is more commonly done with a child and an adult. The liver is split into two unequal parts; the smaller part is given to the child and the larger section to the adult. When a live donor's liver is used, a small portion is taken to be donated, while the donor retains the larger portion.

Bodies from which organs are taken after death are called cadaveric donors. Once they have been pronounced brain dead (irreversible brain damage, no brain activity), their bodies are taken to the operating room, and their viable organs are removed and distributed according to UNOS regulations. Understand that the organ donor has no brain function (brain dead); however, the organs continue to have oxygen-rich blood pumped through them with the help of machines. (i.e., ventilators, intravenous medication, and blood transfusions).

These are commonly referred to as "non-heartbeating donors." These types of donors are still considered very controversial because of the uncontrolled series of events and the possibility of organ damage during the short period of time the organs receive no circulating blood.

Another rare source of organs, especially for pediatric patients, is infants born with anencephaly. These babies are born with little or no brain and often without the top of the skull or spinal cord. They are usually stillborn or survive only a few hours. With ultrasound scanning during pregnancy, the condition can be detected, and often the sad but magnanimous parents make provision to donate the newborn's organs immediately following death.

UNOS and Organ Distribution

The United Network for Organ Sharing is your friend, and you will hear a lot about it during your wait for your new organ.

Organs are selected for patients depending greatly on size and blood type. A potential recipient must receive an organ from a donor with the same, or compatible, blood type, just as in the case of blood transfusions. In addition, the organ has to fit into the recipient, as solid organs are proportional in size (height and ideal body weight) to their bodies. Therefore, a donor five feet, ten inches tall and weighing 165 pounds would not be a good match for a potential recipient listed with UNOS as five-two and weighing 100 pounds. Some data suggest donor and recipient matches should be same-sex matches. Currently, however, gender is not a limiting factor in organ selection.

A government task force published a study on organ procurement and transplantation identifying the need for a system to keep track of donor activity and recipient information. UNOS was formed as a result of that identified need. An agreement was initiated between the government-based task force and Richmond, Virginia–based UNOS. UNOS, in turn, developed the first nationwide distribution system. UNOS keeps track of patients awaiting organs, aids in the placement of organs by maintaining and distributing computerized lists to the regional organ procurement agencies (OPO), set up by geographically identified regions by population. In addition, UNOS tracks transplant center data and reports that data to the appropriate authority. UNOS also assist in developing membership criteria for transplant centers across the U.S. Qualifications for physicians, surgeons, and patient care are mandated by the government through UNOS.

So who gets an organ when one becomes available? How can you be sure this system is fair? When a donor is identified by the hospital staff (i.e., brain dead but maintained on life support), it is a law that the regional organ procurement agency (OPO) be notified. Usually, a nurse coordinator is dispatched to the donor hospital to review the potential donor's medical record, do an examination to evaluate the donor's candidacy, and to ensure that brain death has been determined by appropriate protocols. If indeed the donor qualifies, the donor management coordinator (procurement coordinator) approaches the donor's family about the donation process. Oftentimes the hospital staff has initiated the idea of organ donation as well. The procurement coordinator assumes control of the donor's medical management once the family has agreed to donate and helps them through the grieving process, while the donor is prepared for the operating room. It is at this point a waiting list is run by UNOS to produce a working list of potential recipients, based on blood type, size, and tissue matching. The local transplant center is notified of the potential donation and is offered the organs according to priority. Those transplant centers with patients that are sickest (at the top of the list) are offered the organs first, and the offers continue down the list by priority until a center accepts the organs. Each organ has its own list, and priority on these lists is determined by a organ specific criteria that allows the sickest patients top priority. The only exception to this "sicker gets first pick" rule is with kidneys. Kidneys are offered to centers according to tissue matching (HLA) and are prioritized by waiting time (days) on the list. In other words, if the donor blood type is "A," the UNOS waiting list for "A" kidneys would be run. Tissue matching is done from donor blood and banked recipient (all six antigens are alike), the kidney is offered to that person. If there is no six-antigen match, the next-best match is found and the kidney is offered to the person with the best match who has the most number of days on the list.

Once the organs are accepted by each of the transplant centers (there are usually at least three centers involved), the procurement coordinator begins the laborious task of coordinating operating room schedules, procurement team schedules, and preparing for the actual procurement and transport of the organs from the donor hospital to the accepting centers. Usually at this point, the procurement coordinator and your transplant coordinator (assuming the organ has been allocated to you) have spoken several times and she has notified you of the possibility of your getting your transplant.

Logistics About Organ Distribution

The country is divided under UNOS into eleven regions, and there may be two or three centers of operation in organ procurement and distribution, called organ procurement organizations (OPOs), within each. Right now, organs are distributed geographically, offered first to patients in the community where they are donated, then to patients within the region. There have been several movements by federal and transplant centers alike to change the system of allocation. Steps have been taken by UNOS to ensure equity in the donation process by redefining the list criteria to better recognize the "sickest donors" and to accommodate the needs of less populated and smaller transplant centers so that they may have "equal sharing." The discussions and frequent changes taking place at the government level makes it necessary to say at this time of printing to check with your own transplant coordinator with questions and concerns about specific organ allocation issues. The federal Department of Health and Human Services (HHS) wants to change this allocation procedure so that organs are offered to the sickest patients first, no matter where they live, as long as they have a reasonable chance of survival. Transplant surgeons say the government's proposal would lead to more deaths following transplant because sicker patients would get more organs, and they are less likely to survive. At this writing, the controversy is undergoing discussion and research before a decision is made. By the time you read this book, however, the decision will have probably been made.

Pre-Transplant Medication Program

Talk about custom-made! Not only is your pre-transplant medication program organ specific, it is also patient specific. Before even undergoing transplant, pre-transplant patients must take several medications—each with a different purpose. The dosages of some may be changed from clinic visit to clinic visit, and some will remain constant until transplant. Some medications are given prophylactically, that is, they are given as a preventive measure to protect against infection with harmful bacteria, viruses, or fungi. Patients with gastrointestinal irritation before transplant, due to the medications they are taking or their illness, may be prescribed antiulcer medications. Some patients may be hypertensive or suffer from insomnia and are prescribed medications for these ailments.

MAKING TAKING YOUR MEDICATION EASIER

One new kid on the pharmacy block is the special transplant pharmacy. These special pharmacies work with transplant centers across the United States to provide patients with specialized care. This addition simplifies patients' and support persons' lives immensely. It is an extra security blanket. The pharmacy keeps track of the individual's medication record and notifies the patient if he or she hasn't called for refills. Many transplant pharmacies also have financial advisors who can help with billing questions and with insurance payments. Not all centers use this specialized pharmacy. If yours does not, ask your transplant coordinator for help. He or she can give you information about those that may service your area. Otherwise, you or your caregiver should get to know your local pharmacist and even apprise him or her in advance of your post-transplant needs, so that he or she will be ready for you and your busy caregiver.

A problem many patients (transplant and otherwise) often have is remembering to take their medication. To make matters worse, often patients suffering from liver or kidney failure have encephalopathy: mental confusion caused by a buildup of toxins in the system due to the failure of the organ. This, of course, makes remembering to take one's necessary medications that much harder. There are ways to help patients take control of their own medication regimens and reduce the confusion that may occur.

Some patients use convenient pill containers other than the pharmaceutical ones. For example, many buy small zip-close plastic bags and little paper sticker labels. They put each dosage time on each bag, include the appropriate pills for that time, and put each bag in a larger sealable plastic bag labeled by the day. Other patients suggest electronics parts boxes or even small tackle boxes if you have a lot of medication to manage. Many patients purchase wristwatches with alarms that allow up to five different alarm time settings and then set the alarms at the beginning of the day for all of the times when medication must be taken. This seems to be the most reliable way to remember one's dosing regimen, if you don't forget your watch frequently. Janet identifies a key word here "routine." Incorporate your medication schedule into your routine. Do not attempt to change your routine to fit your medication schedule, since this can lead to frustrations and feeling that medication is controlling your life.

TEAM COMMUNICATION REGARDING YOUR MEDICATION

Both before and after your transplant, you must *never* take any medication that you have not discussed first with your team. This prohibition extends to over-the-counter medications and herbal remedies as well. It extends even to herbal teas, zinc lozenges, and all vitamin and mineral supplements. One dosage of ibuprofen taken for a headache could lead to liver damage in a liver patient. The best rule of thumb with pre- and post-transplant patients and their medications is to be completely open with your team about what you are taking. This is one example of how important communication between you and the coordinator and physician is.

Be up front, too, about what medications you may have stopped taking (though you should never discontinue any medication without first discussing it with your physician)! Perhaps some prescription medication causes an unpleasant side effect. Discuss this matter with your team; usually some adjustment can be made that will bring relief.

Before my transplant, a doctor I visited prior to my liver failure diagnosis had prescribed Zantac (ranitidine hydrochloride) for a peptic ulcer, which, as it turned out, I did not have. I decided then that I'd just stop taking the medication. *Wrong!* As it turned out, I still needed to take the Zantac, and my hepatologist would have prescribed it or another antiulcer drug if I were not already on Zantac. She was not pleased with me.

During the pre-transplant period, you will be visiting the transplant center regularly. These visits are your chance to ask questions, discuss any problems you may have with your medications, discuss your overall health, have blood drawn and tested, and have your condition monitored by the team. If your team finds something troublesome in your blood tests or if you are reporting any problems, you may be asked to come every week or every two weeks for a while. You know that you are doing well when you are not asked to show up for three to four weeks.

Conclusion

You have come, willingly or not, into a circle of amazing people who will, with your help, restore your health. Listen to them; follow their prescriptions and their advice. Use them and the help they have to offer, whether medical, emotional, or financial. Be open to them, while at the same time acting on your own behalf. You have the job of getting well. You are in this adventure with your medical team. Godspeed.

CHAPTER FOUR

Coping As You Wait for Your Transplant

All that you've learned thus far is a lot to digest. Awaiting an organ transplant is no easy thing. It brings lots of life changes and can arouse emotions you never expected, such as fear, guilt, and denial. This chapter offers you ways to deal with these and other emotions and situations you may experience as you await your organ transplant. Some practical matters will also be covered, such as getting your legal affairs in order and utilizing your support system to advantage.

If you were well adjusted in your life before transplant candidacy, you will, in all likelihood, cope well with this new challenge. You may have to dig down deep within yourself to tap into your best resources, but you can do it just as surely as others have before you. The statistics of patient survival in transplantation are on your side. In fact, your wellness is in your hands. How well you fare through this whole venture will depend on your attitude. Janet says that if you ask any recipient what got him or her through transplant, he or she will be quick to reply: a positive attitude, a supportive family and friends, and a great transplant team.

As a transplant patient, I credit my success—medical capabilities notwithstanding—to my absolute insistence that this opportunity would not fail. Put bluntly, I decided that I would not die. It is true that all support that comes your way, medical and personal, is influential in your re-covery; but it is also true that the effort of others is almost wasted if you are not an active participant in your recovery.

Dealing with Various Stressors

When there are stressors present in your life, usually you will experience stress! In other words, it's not all in your head. There are real sources for that feeling that you are being stretched to the end of your emotional rope. Life events, sometimes even happy events like preparing for marriage or a new home, cause stress. Human events are never uncomplicated. Two United States Navy physicians developed a list of life's major stressors. Personal illness or injury is sixth on their list, after death of a spouse, divorce or separation, imprisonment, and death of a close relative.

Learning that you must have a transplant in order to save your life is a big stressor. You are called on to prepare yourself mentally and emotionally for a radical surgical procedure, while you are still trying to cope with the chronic effects of an end-stage organ disease.

PROLONGED HOSPITAL STAYS

The wait is difficult for every candidate for transplantation; it is especially hard for those in need of continuous medical management in the hospital. Heart transplant candidates on assist devices (heart pumps) must wait in the hospital, an unnatural and stressful environment. Oftentimes these types of patients are not as able to participate in some of the coping mechanisms discussed in this book. Indeed, all of their efforts at coping will have to come from within. In the case of kidney-transplant candidates, their wait may be longer, sometimes upward of five years. And their need for dialysis is an additional stress factor in their lives. Patients waiting for livers oftentimes are admitted to the hospital during their wait for a organ due to encephalopathy (altered mental status) or bleeding problems such as gastrointestinal bleeding.

DIMINISHED ENERGY

Diminished energy is a problem for many pre-transplant patients. Heart transplant candidates often must deal with such problems as arrhythmias and shortness of breath on exertion. Kidney patients often suffer from anemia and so have a low tolerance for any kind of exertion. Liver patients, especially those with hepatitis, suffer from chronic fatigue. Nevertheless, some kind of exercise is recommended in order to decrease tension and increase a feeling of well-being.

Janet says:

Don't let your fatigue diminish your desire to do as much as you can to stay as healthy as you can prior to transplant. Take it easy but exercise mentally and physically during the wait. Sometimes you should even push yourself. A person facing transplant should continue to live as normal a life as possible, including continuing to work for as long as possible. Some patients say that they don't know how they'll get up and go to work, but they do much better during the waiting period and postoperatively if their minds and bodies get exercised. If you do have a problem getting to work every day, talk to your employer or human resources department about the possibilities of working fewer hours, part-time, or from home. Increasingly, employers are becoming more sensitive to the needs of those with chronic illnesses.

Exercise ultimately will both increase your energy and relax you. I faithfully followed a walking regimen before my transplant. I suffered from pleural effusion in my lungs, which means that the fluid I retained because of my disease settled around my lungs. When this condition was present, it was exceedingly difficult to breathe without coughing, and I coughed each time I walked a few steps. Usually when my hepatologist modified my diuretics dosage the pressure around my lungs lessened. Even with the chest pressure and coughing, I walked. It is true that I walked with more difficulty, but I walked.

My friend and primary caregiver tells me now that she nearly went out of her mind waiting for me to accomplish the simple task of walking from a door to an elevator. I crept. Outdoors, however, as I walked on the beach in the fresh air, I was able to walk more briskly. I recommend that you walk in the most beautiful and inspiring place you can find. The exercise will make all the difference in regaining your strength post-transplant. Perhaps more important, exercise and your awareness of the beauty of the people and places around you will expand your mind and uplift your spirit. Janet recalls the struggle her husband, David, had with walking. Eight years after transplant, he remembers distinctly the short walk down the drive to the mailbox. He has forgotten many elements of the procedure, but the effort to walk will probably remain in his memory forever.

While exercise should become part of your daily routine, Janet cautions that pre-transplant patients who walk or ride a bicycle should use the same path every day so that their caregivers can know where to find them should they not reach home in a reasonable amount of time. Pace yourself, and remember that you must reserve enough energy to get back home!

CONFUSION

Understandably, confusion caused by encephalopathy, often a result of liver and kidney disease, can be another stressor. The toxicity that causes this problem is managed in liver patients through the use of diuretics and laxatives. In kidney patients, toxicity levels are reduced through dialysis. No liver patient is entirely free of encephalopathy before transplant. He or she may be only mildly encephalopathic, as was I, or in an extreme state of confusion, much as with Alzheimer's disease. The positive difference for liver and kidney candidates is that the condition is reversible once the transplant is undergone. Still, the patient and the caregiver must cope with this stress, if only temporarily. This factor makes waiting for an organ all the more difficult.

The element of confusion will probably be harder on your caregiver than on you. He or she will struggle to allow you some measure of control, though this effort will not come easily. It would be easier for the caregiver to take over all tasks. A bit of oversight and tolerance is required. For example, if the ill member of the household is the one who usually handles the finances, paying the bills, and so on, the caregiver might check the figures and the payments for accuracy but allow the patient to continue the task. The caregiver should make every effort to see that the patient retains his dignity.

Driving is another matter. Janet recalls a patient who thought he could handle driving, until one evening he came to a stoplight. He says that he remembers making a quick mental note to put his foot on the brake, but he hit the gas instead. He went through the red light barely missing two oncoming cars. He immediately pulled over to the side of the road and called for someone to come and drive him home.

As her husband's caregiver, Janet remembers David calling her on the cellphone to tell her that he was driving around the city loop for the second time and didn't know where he was going. "He knew where he was, but had no idea where he was going, and I surely did not know even why he was there!"

The slow response time is the critical issue when deciding whether to drive or not to drive for any pre-transplant patient. Diminished energy results in a slower response time, and certain medication, even if excessive weakness is not present, may slow you down and diminish your reaction time. Consult with your caregiver concerning your degree of confusion and the possible danger of slowed response time. Together, you can select tasks that are both safe and stimulating for you. Driving is always the most difficult thing to give up. It seems to signal our loss of independence. Remember, though, you will never forgive yourself if someone is injured or killed because of your diminished response time. The transplant team takes this so seriously that they will call the state department of motor vehicles and have your license suspended if you continue to drive against medical advice.

One suggestion that helps on days when you seem to be more confused than others is to make lists. If you and your caregiver sit down every evening and make a list of things that need to be done the following day, it will make the day flow more smoothly. Be sure to add even the simplest of tasks—dressing, brushing your hair and teeth, and taking your routine medications. Be sure that you as well as your caregiver know where the list is kept so that you are able to find it the next morning. Janet suggests the refrigerator door.

ROLE REVERSAL

In many homes, when one member of the household is sick, there must be a redistribution of household tasks and chores. More men than women are transplant candidates. Today it is common for both partners in a home to work and to share household tasks. When one member of the household is ill, one partner may have to shoulder more of the financial and household burden than he or she did before the other's illness. In the traditional home, this role reversal may be very stressful for both husband and wife. If the husband is the one who is sick, he may take a leave from work while he awaits his organ and do many of the household tasks, while the wife becomes the chief breadwinner, coming home tired at the end of a workday. The children may not understand. The best way to relieve this stress is to talk about it, preparing everyone in advance for the necessary changes and adjustment. Most transplant patients become candidates while they are still working. This still-normal period offers the opportunity to prepare and plan for the onset of family life changes.

My household consisted of two people, both of whom were working professionals. I was listed as a liver transplant candidate in early August and returned to begin a new semester of teaching in late August. I had every intention of continuing working indefinitely. I did not foresee the complications the pleural effusion I discussed earlier would cause. The increased diuretic dosage would have had me running out of the classroom to the bathroom at erratic times. This complication did not make for effective teaching. My energy was diminishing too, and so I left my academic duties as early as the third week of September. I went on an extended leave of absence. I would not receive my transplant for more than a year and would not return to teaching for almost two years.

I took over all of the household tasks that did not involve heavy work. Since my encephalopathy was mild, I was able to run errands. Yes, with those dangerous slowed responses, I did the grocery shopping, the cooking, the banking, the mailing, and so on. I turned the chore of cooking into a hobby. I watched cooking shows on television. An important change for me was that I couldn't read a lot. I taught literature by profession, but I really couldn't concentrate on the pages of a book. People presume that I worked on my first book, my story of my liver transplant, while I was at home, but I could not. I didn't begin it until after transplant, while I was recovering before going back to work.

I explain my own situation to alert you that things may change a lot, and they may change very quickly. Keep yourself in open communication with your family, caregiver, and entire support team. Discussing role changes will help you make a healthier transition.

FINANCING THE TRANSPLANT

All transplant candidates are invited to contact the staff at the National Transplant Assistance Fund with questions about finances. You may have already found your team, the team social worker, or your insurance plan helpful. This government agency exists to help you with questions about other finance opportunities, including how to apply for medical assistance grants and how to establish a restricted fund with NTAF, which can be used for immediate transplant costs as well as those post-transplant costs that may arise years later—after insurance caps have been reached and other types of coverage have ceased.

When friends and family members ask how they can help financially, refer them to NTAF, who will advise them about fund-raising. Professionals at NTAF will guide the leaders of your fund-raising campaign. Even though a candidate may have adequate insurance, many related expenses are not covered. If you have insurance, your coverage may be limited for transplantation. You may reach caps very quickly and then be left with enormous bills.

Jean Tucke of the NTAF says:

We recommend that all patients awaiting [transplant] consider fund-raising. Many patients at the University of Pittsburgh Medical Center have used fund-raising successfully. One family was able to relocate to Pittsburgh for four months and pay for housing costs with their account. Another patient pays for his post-transplant medications that are not covered by medical insurance.

The transplant candidate with too much time on his hands and some amount of stamina might organize and spearhead his own fund-raising! If the task is too difficult, he or she might at least find some way to contribute his or her efforts to such a campaign.

DOWNTIME

As you await your transplant, you may ultimately have to take time off work, and you may find yourself with little to do. It is easy to worry, and idle time will afford you an opportunity to obsess over all of the negative possibilities. This can, of course, increase your frustration. If you can, fill your time with safe and enjoyable activities and with relaxing meditation/visualization practices.

Choose Hobbies

For me, cooking was a godsend. My challenge as a chef (!) was to adjust the recipes that I copied from my cooking shows to accommodate my low-sodium pre-transplant diet and still make them a culinary delight! Pity my poor housemate-cum-caregiver. Actually, we enjoyed all of my concoctions, and the exercise kept my spirits up.

Some people like to spend some of their downtime traveling and seeing new things. Janet says it's OK to take short trips as long as the transplant center knows where you are and can reach you. The higher you are on the transplant list, however, the more restricted any travel will be. You must be available in the event an organ becomes available for you. When you are accepted as a transplant candidate, you will probably receive a pager. This handy device, familiar to all in the electronic age, will summon you when that life-saving organ is available. Don't leave home without your pager.

I strongly suggest doing things you like to do while waiting. Do light recreational reading, sew, swim, play on the computer, or practice a musical instrument if you are adept. Actually, this time is priceless and is not likely to come again. If you have to stop working or reduce your working time, try to see the downtime as a gift.

MEDITATE AND VISUALIZE

The psychological techniques of meditation and visualization have both proven helpful in improving well-being, diminishing symptoms, and even improving health. Make the mind-body connection. Acknowledge the union of body and spirit and recognize the dimension of the spiritual in health.

There are several different types of meditation, but generally, they involve concentrating on one thing—say, your breathing—and clearing your mind of all other thoughts. With meditation, you should be able to attain a deep level of relaxation very quickly. Many books and courses are available from which you can learn different meditation techniques, with varying degrees of effectiveness for different people.

You can meditate while walking. Concentrate on breathing deeply, from your abdomen, counting steps or breaths. Or focus your attention on the colors and textures around you. Finally you are taking the time to stop and smell the roses.

Visualization, or imagery, is a technique in which you conjure up mental images in order to summon your body's energy to work toward wellness. I practiced visualization as a relaxation technique whenever I was home alone. I would go in my mind from one level of consciousness down deeper to another, while visualizing myself at my favorite scene. That deepest level of consciousness was a serene place where I was most in touch with my self—my spiritual self. I expressed sentiments of hope to myself and to my caregiver and of well-being, asserting that I would be all right and that health and a whole life would return after transplant. I might have called those sentiments an expression of faith and hope.

You, too, might think that I only hoped that I would get better, but I believe that I *determined* my good health. Perhaps my assurance will help you. I determined that I would be OK, and I am! Simplistic? Perhaps. I had an excellent transplant team and unbelievable emotional support, but

ADVICE FROM PEOPLE WHO HAVE BEEN THERE

Though I am a former transplant patient, you might be thinking, "OK, coping with all of these life changes was easy for you, but you are just one person. What about the average transplant patient? How well does he or she cope with waiting for an organ transplant?" Perhaps you will find some words of advice from other transplant patients helpful.

A kidney transplant patient who wrote to me on the Internet (he calls himself the home of Sydney the kidney) had this to say about the worry and anxiety of waiting for an organ transplant: "Worry is like a rocking chair. It gives you something to do, but it doesn't get you anywhere." Another patient found that he gained control by gaining information: "I bought books and read a lot. I felt more in control knowing as much as I did."

Dave, a kidney recipient, relates his difficult story. He has been a paraplegic since the age of five. He had a kidney transplant for his end-stage renal failure that failed almost immediately. He has been waiting since 1994 for a second transplant. Still, he says, "I cope by just going on with life and staying as productive as possible. There may come a day when I can't farm, but I don't worry about things I can't do much about. That's my attitude with transplant and dialysis too. I just don't worry about things I have little or no control over."

Another patient, Michele, who is waiting for a liver, relates to her illness as a journey in which she has, she says,

> been losing things dear to me, but am also able to gain very
> important things as well. With that in mind, I have been able
> to be unapologetically assertive about my need for rest, for
> help at times (which has been a big step for me, being a social

worker and much more comfortable on the other side of the equation), for my needs in general. I have been able to accept the curtailment of energy and of ability to accomplish as much as I need to, the loss of mental clarity and short-term memory, and the loss of body image with much more serenity than I ever could have imagined before.

One heart transplant recipient told her support group:

The thought of once having a garden of my own held me up during those days in ICU and in my lonely room at the transplant clinic after my heart transplant in 1988. I used to lie awake all night listening to the helicopters starting and landing on the roof on the next building. I fantasized about the garden I would have, and I had a special place in mind. I dreamt of buying an old farmhouse from a distant relative of mine. It is by a small, cold lake in the country-side, and it is a beautiful house. I planned all the beds and the paths and trees and bushes I would put in the garden.

Another recipient says of her life after transplant:

I find that one cannot look back but only forward. I plant trees, bushes, and gardens, expecting to watch them grow. I buy material for piles of quilts, collect recipes by the dozens, having no idea where the time to quilt or cook will come from. I try to bake bread often and visit my friends. My house is not clean, but it is a happy home. [I am] not a su-perwoman but an enthusiastic person who cannot stop plan-ning for the future. Don't ever stop planning or reaching for your dreams, whether you are a transplant recipient or just cop-ing with life!

Michele mentions one of the best coping mechanisms of all, humor. Her coordinator, while educating her and other patients about "the list," mentioned that a patient might be bumped from the top by someone with fulminant hepatitis from eating mush-rooms. "At that point I raised my hand and asked where I could buy them!"

Medical researchers form study groups and questionnaires in order to understand patient coping skills. One such study, pub-lished in 1994, was aimed at discovering which coping mecha-nisms had been most helpful for transplant patients, in order to assist caregivers and to minimize stress for future patients. After much studying, research, and assessment, the team concluded that patients coped best by thinking positively, using humor, and continuing to lead a lifestyle that is as normal as possible.

they had to have something to work with. Just imagine how selfish the pa-tient would be who would not do his or her part in the process. This pre-transplant period is not the time to wimp out on everyone or to simply enjoy being the center of attention. You must have a plan. You are prepar-ing for a life-altering experience. Take this time to develop mental, emo-tional, and physical preparedness.

When you feel particularly frustrated during the wait, which is itself the most trying period of the transplant process, talk to a member of your transplant team. Janet suggests that the wait gives you time to build a re-lationship and trust with the team that will help see you through. This team will be a part of your life for a long time. As an illustration of this fact, make a list of the people who have come into your life—your team, friends you have met along the way, other transplant recipients, those that wait along with you for the gift of life.

FALSE ALARMS

The entire waiting time is both stressful and frustrating. Sometimes the stress and anxiety can be further exacerbated by false alarms. Sometimes a patient is contacted and told that the team has found a suitable organ and to come to the center. Naturally, the patient's anxiety and anticipation run high. You arrive, perhaps begin undergoing the preparation for surgery, and then are told that the organ is defective and you must return home to continue waiting. These "false alarms" do occur. I was paged four times before I actually received my donated organ. Three of those four times I entered the hospital and went through the protocol—I was x-rayed, showered, was given enemas, and had my heart monitored and my vital signs registered. After several hours of waiting and fasting, I was told to get dressed and go home. I left the hospital with mixed feelings. I was relieved that I wasn't facing a life-threatening procedure yet but disappointed that all the waiting wasn't over.

You can be sure that the transplant team has your best interests in mind when choosing an appropriate organ. In this time of organ shortages, and with the ever-changing allocation rules, the team may pass on organs offered for one reason or another several times before the right one is accepted. Organs from "marginal donors" are so classified because they carry risk factors that are not necessarily contraindications for use but that may make them less than perfect for use. Such an organ may be from an older donor or a donor who has tested positive for hepatitis (meaning that he or she was *exposed* to the virus, not necessarily that he or she *has* the virus.) These donors are OK for use in recipients who test positive as well, but are not ideal in a situation in which the recipient has never been exposed to hepatitis.

Before death, the donor's blood pressure may not have been high enough to ensure that blood is circulating through the organ for too long a time. These organs are used for patients who are critically ill and not expected to live without immediate transplant. As the number of patients waiting for organ transplant continues to rise, while the size of the donor pool remains the same, transplant teams are forced to expand their criteria to accept some of these marginal donors.

Usually a patient is not called until it is the time for transplant, but sometimes these false starts do occur. The organ is examined very carefully by the surgeon for any defects. If the organ is flown in from another place, the surgeon may not have had the opportunity to examine it closely until it reaches the home facility.

Once you get that call, you can expect the team to keep you and your family informed on any delays or changes in plan. False alarms are unavoidable and are frustrating for everyone, including the transplant team. It is easy to forget that the team has worked to coordinate the organ procurement, has traveled to a distant hospital to assess the organ, and has coordinated your admission and preoperative care. They are frustrated as well.

Try to look at the situation positively. The organ is rejected in your best interest. No one—not the team or the patient—wants to begin the difficult transplant process with a defective organ. Sometimes any organ is welcome, but only as a temporary measure to save a dying patient in full organ failure.

BEING PASSED OVER ON THE LIST

Another source of frustration and stress is to watch as someone who was placed on the list after you is transplanted before you. Because of all of the variables involved in an organ match, this pass-over will probably occur. I was passed over for a woman with my same blood type. The fact was not called to my attention, but candidates always have an active grapevine. The woman was a little older than me and very encephalopathic. I didn't feel any frustration or resentment. I just kept believing that everything would be all right.

It's OK to hope that another organ will become available. A lot of people feel guilty about feeling this way—that it is as if they are hoping someone will die. Janet and David recall their response to a breaking news story about a number of people involved in an unfortunate hostage situation during David's pre-transplant period: "We both jumped up from our chairs and checked the batteries in the beeper!" You cannot feel guilty for these situations. Yes, unfortunately, someone must die in order for you to receive your organ, but that person was good enough in life to choose to donate it—to give the gift of life in his or her death.

FINANCIAL PROBLEMS

Among the biggest stressors that accompany the wait for an organ are financial matters. How are you going to pay for everything? Medical insurance covers only so much of the cost of transplant. After that, it seems like you are pretty much on your own. And while you may have enough money to cover some of the additional costs of transplant, the rest of your life or the lives of those in your family have not stopped. You still have other expenses to consider outside of your health problems. All of your money cannot go to the cost of your transplant.

Often finances are the reason people continue to work even when they are really no longer capable. Janet's husband, David, kept working for almost nine months until he reached his twenty-year retirement with the Houston Fire Department. How would you like to have him driving a fire truck to save your home?! A good bit of the coping with the time before transplant just requires common sense. If it is safer and healthier to stop work, you should stop.

The social services department at the transplant center can help in connecting you to government assistance available to end-stage organ disease patients. Usually Social Security Insurance (SSI) is available for long-term disability. One cannot start to receive Social Security Disability until six months after the date that the Social Security Administration (SSA) determines that one became disabled. According to a pamphlet published by the Social Security Administration, "You will be considered disabled if you are unable to do any kind of work for which you are suited and your disability is expected to last for at least a year. . . . The program assumes that working families have access to other resources to provide support during periods of short-term disabilities." Social Security Disability pays cash benefits to those considered disabled. Benefits continue until a person is able to work again on a regular basis, and a number of work incentives are available to ease the transition back to work. Some employers maintain long-term disability policies for their employees. With my university's disability policy and SSI, I received 60 percent of my pre-illness salary until transplant and for one year after.

The important thing to remember is to begin financial planning as soon as you learn that you will need a transplant. The transplant family that plans ahead does best in coping with finances.

LOSS OF CONTROL

Pre-transplant patients often feel as though they have no control over their own lives. They feel as though they must check each element of their lives with the transplant team. Their abilities and activities are limited to begin with, and to make things worse, anything new that they may feel that they can do and would like to try must first be okayed by someone else. This can be a significant source of stress and frustration. The loss of control will be an irritation both before and for a time after transplant.

I recall a time when I really got fed up. I wanted to take a short trip just for a change. It seemed that I had been hanging around at home to no good end forever. I waited for my transplant for fourteen months. At the time I wanted to go away, I was at the top of the list for my blood type, so my surgeon denied my excursion. My liver could have become available while I was gone, and I'd be too far away. Now it wasn't as if I wanted to get lost in the desert or the mountains; there were telephones where I was headed. But my transplant surgeon said no. No meant no. I coped with my disappointment by combining tantrum and humor. I began sending postcards to the team—from the city in which I lived, where the transplant medical center was also located. Since it is a tourist town, I could select postcards of my own condominium, an antiquated building on the hospital grounds, a sky shot of a gnarly nearby freeway, and so on. Later, post-transplant, when I was writing my book on my liver transplant, I had access to my medical files. Sure enough, there were the postcards, saved for whatever reason. Proof of mental confusion? Or a good coping style with humor?

Janet insists that, unfortunately, the more control the team has, the better prepared for transplant the patient will be. Sometimes the patient is admitted to the hospital simply so that the team can have control over his or her proper diet, rest, and medications. There comes a time when the patient and family just have to trust the team. A careful balance has to be maintained. If the patient is "babied" too much before transplant, he or she may not easily comply with the regimen after transplant.

The best antidote for not being in control of so many facets of one's life is to have control over a few. Your attitude, your outlook, your evenness of temperament, your optimism, and your resolve are within your control. Your inner self is yours to protect and strengthen. You can also control your compliance. Nobody can make you take your medication or moderate your fluid intake or eat less salt. Your worst enemy, or your greatest ally, in all of this can be "the committee in your head," which can rationalize like crazy. It all comes down to this: Do you want to live? Then don't jeopardize your chance.

DENIAL

Sometimes, patients may begin to wonder if a transplant is even necessary. Though they've been accepted as transplant candidates, they really don't feel sick. They can carry on normal activities. They begin to wonder: "Do I really need an organ transplant?" This apparent feeling of wellness occurs because the illness has been present for so long that the body compensates for a while. It compensates for a lack of energy or a lack of concentration. Thus the patient doesn't realize how sick he or she is. A patient may go for years before seeking medical attention. Once you receive some management for your disease you may indeed begin to feel better. Almost inevitably, at some time before transplant, the patient will ask a team member with eagerness and naïve hopefulness, "Do I still have to have a transplant?" "Yes" will be the resounding reply. As long as the patient alternates between "Yes, I must have a transplant, and it will be successful in restoring my health," and "Maybe I have become well enough that I won't need a transplant after all," he will suffer stress from the contradictory impulses. His peace of mind, as well as the efficacy of his preparation, depends on a full commitment to a successful transplant. Anything less works against him psychologically.

ANXIETY

Anxiety is a common feeling in the pre-transplant period. This transplant is your only option for return to a normal life. A million "what ifs" can plague you while you wait. What if an organ doesn't become available for you in time? What if I'm next on the list and I suddenly catch a virus or some other type of infection, making me too ill to undergo surgery? What if something goes wrong during the surgery? What if my body rejects the transplanted organ? What if there are complications? Will I survive? What if, what if, what if . . .

In addition, sometimes the pager creates anxiety. Someone may dial a wrong number, inadvertently beeping you. Sometimes active weather with thunderstorms and lightning causes the pager to beep. Janet once worked as a coordinator in Texas, where thunderstorms are frequent in the early spring and summer. She says she got to the point that she could predict the course of the storm by the calls she received from the candidates whose beepers were false-alarming. She had candidates scattered from the lower valley of Texas to the border of Louisiana. As the storm traveled from west to east, the candidates called from their respective locations. Thunderstorms along the Gulf Coast meant sleepless nights for the coordinator, as well as the candidates.

Liver, heart, and lung patients generally suffer from the most anxiety, as their conditions are generally the most life-threatening. Most kidney and pancreas patients can continue to rely on dialysis and insulin, respectively, while they await their transplants, though their quality of life is not optimal.

Relaxation is the key to dealing with anxiety. There are several relaxation techniques available to you. Meditation is among the most popular and perhaps the most effective. Again, there are several books on meditation. Check a few out of the library and try to find which technique works best for you.

There are several herbal preparations and supplements that are supposed to promote relaxation. It is important to remember: *Do not ingest anything, even an herbal tea blend, without first checking with your team.* Even the most seemingly innocuous preparation can have ill effects on the transplant process if your doctors are unaware that you are taking it.

One of the handiest relaxation techniques is always available to you: a soak in a nice warm bath. My hepatologist recommended this to me for relaxation at bedtime to help with insomnia. You may want to "dress up" the bathroom for this. Light candles and place scented products such as fragrant essential oils, incense, and potpourri throughout the room (check with the team before adding anything to the bath water). It is believed that scents can affect your mood. The science of aromatherapy says that scents that induce relaxation include lavender, jasmine, chamomile, rose, bergamot, ylang ylang, and clary sage. You can add any of these essential oils to a vaporizer or diffuser, or you can boil a pot of water and add several drops, letting the steam fill your room.

Massage can be helpful in relieving anxiety, as well. Perhaps a loved one would offer you a relaxing back and shoulder massage. Even better, treat yourself to a professional massage!

Diana L. Ajjan of the Natural Medicine Collective, a consortium of health-care practitioners devoted to natural healing, suggests deep breathing as a way of relieving anxiety and stress. "Deep breathing relaxes your body and mind so that you can examine sour negative thoughts and replace them with more positive ones," she says. To practice deep breathing, lie down on the floor with your knees bent and feet apart. Be sure that your back is flat on the floor and that you are fully relaxed. With one hand on your abdomen, inhale slowly and deeply through your nose, taking the breath into your stomach so that your hand feels it rise. Your chest should move slightly along with your abdomen. Gently exhale through your nose. Practice doing this until it feels comfortable. Once you become proficient, breathing this way can help relax you whenever necessary.

FEAR

Anxiety is a generalized feeling of dread. Fear is a more specific feeling that is directed toward something: fear of dying, fear of complications, fear of not getting an organ in time, fear of the unknown, of how things will work out. No matter how hard they may try, the members of the team cannot tell you exactly what the transplant process will be like. You may fear that you will never be able to do the things you want to do again.

Fear is a perfectly natural and healthy emotion to experience as you await your transplant. Of course, it is not a comfortable feeling at all, and over time the stress that fear causes could affect your health. So how do you cope with being afraid, and is there any way of making those feelings go away?

Utilizing relaxation techniques is one way of dealing with your fear. Any of the relaxation techniques mentioned on pages 58–59 may be useful in helping relieve the tension that fear may bring. Talking is also a good way to relieve both anxiety and fear. Sometimes just expressing your fears out loud is helpful in allaying them, if only a little bit. You may find it difficult to discuss such big fears as fear of dying with loved ones. You may worry about upsetting them or increasing their fears. In such cases (or perhaps even in addition to talking with friends and loved ones) it may be useful to talk to a professional counselor—especially if your fear becomes all-consuming. This can be a traumatic and stressful period for you to go through. You don't have to try to cope all alone.

Systematic desensitization is another useful method for coping with fear . . . and perhaps eliminating it altogether. With systematic desensitization, you focus on your fear. In a relaxed environment, you play that worst-case scenario out in your head. Then as the anxiety and tension build up, you stop imagining the fearful situation and relax, utilizing one of the relaxation techniques on pages 58–59 if necessary. Once you have completely calmed down, try again. Over time, this process can help you desensitize yourself to your fears. It can be even more effective under the direction of a therapist or some other mental health professional. Try it.

GUILT

Guilt is another common emotion pre-transplant patients feel, perhaps because a person must die in order for you to receive their needed organ or because of the extreme generosity of living donors. Many transplant patients will also feel a kind of guilt post-transplant, for perhaps the same reasons. A very competent psychotherapist told me once that feelings are just that—feelings. They should not precipitate guilt. You have not willed them or acted on them. They are just fleeting thoughts. It is true that in my support group we anticipated holidays as a fertile opportunity for organ donation. We would joke about the state raising the speed limit! Admittedly a bit dark. I always kept in mind that my receiving an organ would not *cause* the death of another. The two events are entirely separate manifestations of life on this earth.

Candidates with alcoholic liver disease are hit the hardest with feelings of guilt. They feel that they are responsible for their disease; they did this to themselves by their abuse of alcohol or drugs. Sober and on their way to transplant, there is often a period in which they think that they are not deserving of such a gift. Those feelings are best worked out with a psychologist or a social worker. Often it is helpful to suggest that one should make every effort to live for one's family, whom one may have injured in the past, by being a kinder, gentler, renewed person.

Janet finds that guilt becomes more a component of the waiting experience the longer the wait. Even patients whose disease originated in a way they had no control over may feel guilty when another patient from their support group dies before receiving an organ. The team becomes very vigilant when such a death occurs. Chemically dependent patients are watched especially for signs of depression and guilt. Often they do not, out of a sense of self-worthlessness, seek help.

DEPRESSION

Stress, anxiety, fear, and guilt can all lead to depression if not caught in time. These emotional and psychological problems are the reason the transplant team includes a psychotherapist. All pre-transplant patients become anxious and "blue" at times. Most are healthy emotionally; they just find themselves in an extreme set of circumstances and need coping skills. It is the rare patient who is clinically depressed. (Indeed, if depression is a preexistent condition, it may be a contraindication to transplantation. Real depression threatens to exceed the patient's coping capacity.) Peter C. Whybrow, a psychiatrist, says:

> *Throughout life, human beings strive for meaning and for a stable future in which change can be predicted and controlled to serve a personal destiny. Transient episodes of sadness and depression are*

*ubiquitous, and important points of emotional reference as we navi-
gate the complexities of everyday life. These moments of common
experience are entirely distinct, however, from the illness of melancholia. The roots of serious melancholic depression grow slowly over
years and are usually shaped by many separate events, each of
which combines in a way unique to the individual.*

The average transplant patient is not trapped in a depression. He or
she is more reasonably reacting to some very real stressors that at times
seem overwhelming. Dr. Whybrow believes that we can talk our way into
depression and we can talk our way out. If the feeling of melancholia per-
sists, it might be wise to do some of that talking with the resident psychiatrist.

The physician will probably not administer antidepressant medication
pre-transplant. If antidepressants are not metabolized properly, they can
lead to a rapid toxicity in the system of an end-stage organ failure patient.

SEXUAL DYSFUNCTION

It is likely that the pre-transplant patient will experience sexual dysfunction. Some of this dysfunction comes from diminished energy. If you feel
tired all the time, sex and intimacy may look like just one big hurdle in the
course of an exhausting day. Desire may be reduced because of medication. Some diuretics cause erectile problems in men. Medicines may also
cause vaginal dryness in women. When a kidney patient dialyzes, he or
she may be too tired for sex later. Symptoms of end-stage renal disease,
such as uremic toxicity, may cause loss of the sex drive. In liver patients
the usual hormonal functions are altered by the disease. Heart patients are
even encouraged by the team not to have sexual relations. Most cannot
anyway because of chronic shortness of breath. This all sounds very grim,
doesn't it?

There is irony in this situation. Of all times in the life of a relationship
when both partners need each other's comfort, it is pre-transplant, as it is
in any other serious illness. The overburdened caregiver needs to feel ap-
preciated in order to go on. The patient needs the healing, reassuring

touch of the other. Again, a real generosity is demanded of both. It does not take much energy to cuddle, to caress, to soothe, and to hold and kiss. If the couple does not have sexual expectations, then if arousal comes or does not come, there is still an enjoyment and a comfort in the other's body. It may be that there are some surprises in all this!

Of course, communication is always necessary. There is actually a lot to talk about in this new adventure and new feelings to share. In all likelihood, a couple has never grappled so deeply and keenly with issues of life and death. A new bond is formed, a keepsake of the heart, regardless of the organ affected. The good news is that, for most patients, the dysfunction is reversed at transplant. One could laugh and say that you are getting more than one organ transplanted!

Using Your Support System

All this brings us naturally to the subject of the all-important support person and group—your "system," in transplant jargon. Janet reminds us that the team examines not just the patient but also his or her support system. The support system pre-transplant is twofold: the personal immediate caregiver, usually the spouse or significant other, and the support group at the center. In addition, there is Internet access to information and support.

YOUR PERSONAL CAREGIVER

On the personal level, the support person is so important that some centers will not transplant a patient who has no one to rely on, because the team anticipates a poor outcome. Janet insists that the transplant procedure is harder on the caregiver before and after transplant than on the patient. She tells families that they are being transplanted also. "We are not only changing the recipient's lifestyle, but the family's as well."

Janet puts on her caregiver hat to say:

Waiting for a liver for David was probably the most difficult time I have ever been through in my life. When he had to retire from the fire department and became so encephalopathic that he couldn't find his way out of the back yard, I was solely responsible for bringing in the income and taking care of two teenaged boys, two cocker spaniels, a house, and all it involved. He had frequent visits to the hospital due to complications of end-stage liver disease. He had difficulty sleeping at night, so I did as well. Often, I would get up and go to work with only two or three hours of sleep. David had been wandering around the house most of the night. I feared he would turn on the gas stove and forget to turn it off or wander down the street only to become lost. I tried to keep his life as normal as possible because I knew how difficult it was for him.

She repeats: "One thing caregivers need to realize is that, unlike confusion due to age, patients with end-stage organ disease become confused and disoriented but they still have a reasonably rational idea of what is going on. They don't understand why they are doing what they do."

Another burden is added to the caregiver's role when the patient changes his or her personality. He or she may become quite obstinate and argue over anything. The patient's frustrations are taken out on the most accessible person, the caregiver. The caregiver feels as if he or she is giving all he or she can give. These stresses are hard on a marriage. If the relationship is a strong one, it may not only survive but thrive, but if the partnership was rocky already before an illness, it may crash and burn. Five percent of marriages end in divorce post-transplant. We take this matter up later, but most experts agree that in these cases the disease may have masked problems of another nature. There is no doubt that the support person needs some support—his or her own "system." The caregiver may need to take a day off, do something special for himself or herself. An extended family and/or a circle of friends can be of inestimable help to the helper!

YOUR SUPPORT GROUP

This institutional group is usually organ specific and meets once or twice a month. The team coordinator and/or the social worker is responsible for the agenda of the group's meeting. Sometimes there is a formal presentation of information about transplant, and always there is exchange among members, anecdotal and animated. The session is an opportunity to give and receive information about transplant.

Without any question, the caregivers of encephalopathic patients, those with end-stage renal and liver failure, have it the hardest. Fortunately, the support group is there for them, too. They also attend—or, in some centers, have their own group—and can tap into the resources and suggestions available from the team, other "senior" caregivers, and recipients. A woman sitting in on a small group of caregivers at a recent support group commented: "He was the biggest pain in the ass I have ever been around for the first few weeks after discharge! There! I feel much better for having said that. Thank you for listening!" Patients and recipients have the common goal of surviving transplant happily and healthfully. They can rely on each other's strengths, sometimes realizing that others are having an even more difficult time than they. Sometimes an identification, a connection, is established, a special relationship develops, and patients help each other. Some support groups are developing mentoring programs that seem to work well. Check with your transplant coordinator for support groups at your center. Mark the meetings on your calendar, and go as often as you can. You will not be sorry.

ON-LINE SUPPORT

In this Internet age there are several sites where patients and their caregivers can get and post information. Some are organ specific, and some, such as Medline, presume a level of medical sophistication. The most active on-line support group, and it is monitored by physicians, is *TRNSPLNT@WUVMD.WUSTL.EDU* (for organ transplant recipients and anyone else interested in the issues). Some of the advice we are passing along to you in this book was offered by members of this group in answer to our request for coping strategies that worked.

TENDING TO LEGAL AFFAIRS

It is a good idea to get your legal affairs in order during the pre-transplant period. The center probably has an ethicist on the staff who can assist you if you do not have a lawyer.

Actually, a lawyer is not necessary for living wills. The form is simple and easy to complete and it simply assists you in determining, while you are alive, how you wish to be treated at the time of your death. Do you want to be on extraordinary life support, should you be brain dead? You might think, too, about a power of attorney for a loved one, either a testament allowing for health decisions, should you be unable to make them, or a power that extends to all of your affairs and is placed with your primary caregiver, with a copy to the transplant team. These are simple human matters that, more than depressing the patient, can liberate him or her. The best way to approach surgery is in peace and with a vital hope.

There may be other legal issues you need to resolve even while undergoing evaluation for candidacy. These issues should be declared to the transplant team. Perhaps you have an outstanding traffic warrant? It will be hard to deal with these issues later. The team may not be willing to take on a court battle so that you can be listed. Janet recalls one fellow who was scheduled to do time for a felony. Unfortunately, he had forgotten to mention this fact to the transplant team during evaluation, and he was on the transplant list! She recalls the call in the middle of the night from the sheriff. When he was finally arrested, the candidate instantly gave him her card!

Conclusion

Waiting is in and of itself the chief stress factor for pre-transplant patients. One is entirely out of control of one's future, subject to a nonverifiable list. Human beings do not like ambiguity, and we want things settled and are not comfortable in a slow-moving line. The great stress is the matter of whether or not an organ will be found in time. This is the fear of impending death.

One can be an active participant in extending one's life, however. One can exercise to the extent possible. Such exercise can range from "chair exercises," to brisk walking, depending on one's energy level. Any type of exercise helps reduce swelling, maintain muscle strength, and relieve anxiety and depression.

You can actively preside over your nutrition, controlling sodium and fat intake (and in some prescribed cases, sugar).

You can make every available effort to communicate with your support group peers, your medical personnel, and your home caretakers, especially your significant other. To avoid isolation and depression, you may extend your support to others in the group, facilitating communication by an exchange of phone numbers, for example, or helping a particularly sad or lonely fellow patient.

You should continue any creative skill that is yours, perhaps keeping a writing journal or photo journal of your transplant history or painting images as an artistic mirror of your soul state. You must be self-determined and enlightened, asking questions at every opportunity and focusing on your own agenda for the sake of your good attitude and healing. Everything is *not* out of your control.

You can invent your own plan for coping—an intelligent, personalized one. What you must do is give up or turn your wellness over entirely to others. You should be the one most motivated toward your own healing. You are about to receive an awesome gift, someone else's living organ. You will never feel entirely worthy of it, but neither should you feel unworthy. You can prepare for it, and you can begin to do, in a decided, committed way, some optimistic, generous planning for your future use of the gift of life.

PART TWO

Transplant

CHAPTER FIVE

The Wait Is Over

The call comes. This time the telephone call from your coordinator is not about a change in your medications or a missed appointment. This time he or she says, "We have an organ for you, and it looks good." This is it! What next?

Before any information is given, the coordinator will probably first ask how you are feeling. "Have you had any symptoms in the last week or so of concern, such as fever, night sweats, nausea, vomiting, diarrhea?" If all answers are no, then the coordinator will let you know that there may be an organ available for you. The call doesn't guarantee a transplant, though. A lot still depends on the organ's condition and on yours. If you are in good health, though, the coordinator will tell you where you need to go and when you need to be there. He or she will also caution you not to eat or drink anything after a certain time, usual protocol when anesthesia is going to be administered.

The overall condition of the organ may be known only after the transplant surgeon has had a chance to examine it thoroughly. Theoretically, then, a candidate may be told to come to the transplant center and begin preparing for surgery, only to find out that the organ is not acceptable. It might have a slight defect, invisible to the naked eye. Any serious defects would be known at the time the organ is offered, and the organ would be refused by the candidate's team before a recipient is called.

When you receive the call, you will be told when you should come in to the center hospital. You will probably receive a second call, after the surgeon has seen the organ, and you will be assured that you should be ready. The phone message and your time of arrival are contingent on geographic circumstances. You may be at some distance from the center and the organ, in which case, you will be told to come to the center as soon as possible, even before the surgeon has procured the organ.

YOU ARE READY!

The call notifying you that an organ is available is often scary. Almost without exception, patients ask themselves one last time: "Do I really need a transplant?" This question is born out of the months of fear, anxiety, and other emotions one experiences while awaiting an available organ. The question has some logic behind it, as crazy as it seems. In many cases, a patient is feeling better—physically and emotionally—at this point than when he or she first met the transplant team. Janet asks that you keep in mind that you are feeling as well as you are because of the considerable time and effort you and the transplant team have put into preparing you and your family for this moment. Now you must trust them. For a while, they will be largely in control of your life and your destiny. They are ready, and so are you!

Preparing for the Hospital

You may be tempted to bring a trunk full of personal items with you to the hospital in attempts to make your stay as comfortable as possible; but resist the urge. After surgery, you will be moved directly to the intensive care unit (ICU), where you will remain for three or four days, and there is little room in the ICU for your belongings. By the same token, do not leave at home important items that may on the surface seem to be inconsequential. For example, if you wear glasses—even just for reading—bring them, and a case, with you. Your family member or friend can hold on to them until you awaken.

After my surgery, I wanted to communicate with the doctors but was intubated and could not speak. They gave me a pen and paper so that I could write what I wanted to say, but as I tried to write, I realized that I did not have my glasses and could not see to write. I never thought that I would need my glasses immediately following surgery, but I did.

If you wear dentures, wear them to the hospital, and bring the case. If you live some distance from the center and family members cannot make quick runs between the center and home, you may want to bring sleepwear, a robe, and slippers for later on the ward. Presumably the recipient will wear home what he wore to the hospital. Toiletries will, for the most part, be supplied by the hospital in that famous "kit" that the patient pays for. He or she could bring along anything of a personal nature that is important to him, e.g., makeup, a special cologne. With all of these personal items, keep in mind that the recipient will not return to the same room he had before the surgery. He will spend a few days to a week in the Surgical Intensive Care Unit, where there is no storage, before going to still another room on the ward.

HELPFUL TIPS ON DECISIONS TO MAKE BEFORE SURGERY

While you are in the hospital awaiting your surgery, it is a good opportunity to speak with the coordinator about any cultural or religious needs before or after surgery. For example, some women of Middle Eastern background may require that their heads be covered, even on the way to surgery. A Roman Catholic might request the Sacrament for the Sick be administered before surgery. The team tries to accommodate requests that are reasonable.

VISITORS

It is good idea for the patient and his or her family to decide on any visitor restrictions before surgery. Certainly the ICU is not the place for socializing. A patient's stay there is a critical time. Some time must pass before the new recipient is considered to be stable. The patient's family may certainly appreciate the support of visitors, but such visitors should stay out of the ICU. Each transplant center has its own visiting policies. In some, only immediate family members are allowed. Know your hospital's policies in advance to cut down on confusion. If any visitors, for whatever reason, are unwelcome, then do not add them to your list. Medical personnel are adept at screening visitors. Your team is still there to support you. Talk to them. Put your trust in the transplant team. They are putting their knowledge and experience to work in directing your care. Remember that you did your homework in finding this team, and they have not let you down yet. They will get you through this difficult time. The transplant team has a vested interest in you and your newly transplanted organ. Much like a new set of parents, the transplant team is very protective.

Small children, and perhaps even impressionable teenagers, should not be allowed to visit in the ICU in the postoperative period. The children may have a hard time dealing with what they see: multiple lines, tubes, and drains. They may be overwhelmed. Janet has had recipients' children say that they wish that they had never gone in; it was too scary. No one wants to leave that impression on the children.

A member of my support group showed a picture of himself taken by his wife in ICU. I had just begun attending the support group. A lasting horrific impression was made on me. I had not been really afraid until I saw that picture. Of course, when it was my turn, I realized that he had felt fine when the picture was taken and that most of the lines and tubes are removed very quickly. He was celebrating with a Pepsi. I still wouldn't recommend the picture as an ad for the product!

TELEPHONE CALLS

Be sure that you make a list of phone numbers of the people you want notified once the surgery is over for your family member or friend who accompanies you to the hospital. This will ease the stress placed on this person as he or she tries to notify everyone of your status. Your caregiver would be wise to bring lots of change for the pay phone or a phone card.

Janet suggests that candidates buy a twenty-dollar phone card and pack it along with the few items needed for the preliminary trip to the hospital. Often pay phones are the only telephones available in the ICU waiting room. Cellphones are often discouraged inside the hospital because they interrupt the telemetry of some of the hospital equipment. The caregiver would have to go outside to get good cellphone reception. Many have found that it is easier to have their loved one call a designated few, who then can call others. This helps relieve some of the stress placed on the accompanying loved one, who may be exhausted.

Conclusion

There are so many things to think about when one enters the hospital for an indefinite period of time. Being as prepared as possible will help ease the stress that such an occasion causes. It is good to think of the little things, because even small details are irritating when one is facing such a big thing as organ transplantation. Bring very few personal items; your caregiver can supply more later. Take care of social relations, such as phone calls and visitors, so that nothing of that kind will bother you later. Remember, too, in the midst of the flurry, that the phone call from the co-ordinator will prompt you to act as if this is *the* call, but you should be prepared to accept that the organ might not be just right, and you may have to repeat the drill on a later occasion. You'll have it down pat when the real time comes.

CHAPTER SIX

Transplanting Your New Organ

A great deal has been going on behind the scenes in attempts to get you the right organ safely and in a timely manner while you prepared for your hospital stay and surgery. Now that an organ is available for you, all that you and your caretaker have to do is go to the hospital. The moment that you have been waiting and preparing for is upon you. Of course you've got a few butterflies, but by this time you also have the utmost confidence in your transplant team and in yourself. You have been a member of this team; now you will use the education and skills you have attained to put yourself at ease. This just may be one of the most important episodes in your life.

This chapter outlines what you can expect after you have received the call from your coordinator. We will discuss not only what you will be doing but also what is going on behind the scene, what the transplant team is doing in preparation for your transplant.

Getting the Organ to Your Hospital

There are several steps involved in getting the chosen organ to the operating room for your surgery. First it must be removed from the donor, then treated and transported.

PROCURING THE ORGAN FROM THE DONOR

The organ is procured by the local organ procurement organization (OPO) from the donor hospital. The transplant center's coordinator will arrange the transportation of the organ. The OPO representative arrives at the donor's hospital and makes sure that it was indeed the desire of the donor or his or her family to offer the organs for transplant. The transplant center's team is often involved in the procurement—sometimes along with members of other transplant teams. Some procurement procedures are shorter than others, depending on the number of organs the family has consented to donate. Sometimes the family does not want to donate the heart or the corneas. The heart is often perceived as the seat of the emotions, the physical entity from which love flows. The corneas of the eyes are so identified with the soul of the donor that they, likewise, may be restricted from donation. The OPOs must honor the donor and the donor family's wishes. In cases in which the donor was sick for a long time, the lungs are often declared inadequate by the OPO coordinator, because of reliance on a ventilator.

Geography may delay the transplant. If the organ is procured from several or more miles away, the time of transplant may be pushed back to accommodate the arrival time. Often the transplant coordinator has to tell the patient and family that there is a delay. The delay does not suggest that anything is awry. All of the needs of multiple transplant centers must be accommodated. The procured organs may be dispatched to several centers. When the appropriate surgeons are in place at the donor hospital, procurement begins. The complete evacuation of organs usually takes three to four hours.

TREATMENT OF THE PROCURED ORGAN

The organs are cooled and flushed of any donor blood that may be in them. Then they are permeated with a special very cold, rich solution that will preserve them. They are placed with ice and more of the solution in sterile bags, which are then placed in ordinary insulated coolers. They are taken to the respective recipient hospitals by members of the transplant teams. During a procurement procedure the heart is removed first (with the lungs if they are going as well) and the cardiac team leaves the remainder of the procedure to the team or teams taking the liver, kidneys, and pancreas. The rational behind this involves timing. A heart and lungs only have a short period of time they can stay outside the body without blood and oxygen circulating through them (ischemic time), usually 4 to 6 hours. The liver and pancreas usually require perfusion prior to 16 to 18 hours, while kidneys are less likely to be damaged and can stay on ice for 24 to 48 hours.

TRANSPORT OF THE ORGAN

In some instances, as with kidneys when the need for transplant is not immediate, organs are taken to airports and shipped by commercial airline to the airport closest to the transplant facility. The organs are either accompanied by flight attendants or are placed in the captain's quarters. They are never just placed in the baggage compartment. Janet admits, however, that one time an organ was presumed "lost," but she eventually found it going round and round at the baggage claim area. It was on the belt in a box marked "Human Organs for Transplantation" in bright orange lettering!

Generally, the organs come back to the center with the surgeon who removed them. This method is best because it affords control of the organ and the schedule. It offers a better estimate of the time for beginning the transplant procedure. In addition, if the transplant surgeon procures the organ, he or she can see how the organ sets in the donor body and whether or not there were any irregularities there, for example, in the vasculature (blood vessel network). This opportunity offers the surgeon a better idea of how the organ will fit into the recipient. In addition, transplant centers have different techniques for procurement and so are more comfortable with procuring their own donor organs. Occasionally they can count on surgeons at the donor site to follow the transplant surgeon's protocol.

The Transplant Procedure

Once the organ is on its way back to the transplant center, the candidate is prepared for surgery: an enema is administered, the patient is told to shower, the heart is monitored one last time, and an IV line is begun for hydration and later for anesthesia. Rarely, but possibly, the patient may get this far and be told that the organ is defective and to go home. This extraordinary chain of events happened to me the first time I was called.

This time spent outside the operating room can be full of anxiety for the candidate. Depending on his or her frame of mind, the patient might say goodbye to his loved ones thinking that this might be the last time he or she will see them. I have said earlier that I had decided I was not going to die. I recommend this effective, if somewhat naïve, optimism. Usually the family, especially the husband or wife, or the person closest to the candidate, is allowed to remain with him until he is rolled into the operating room. The team acknowledges that this is a life-threatening surgery. The family will want some quiet time perhaps to pray together.

When it is decided that all systems are go, you will be wheeled in the operating room on a gurney. Once you are in there the anesthesia is begun, and the next thing you know you are waking up what seems like minutes later.

Regardless of expectations, the transplant surgery is tricky. The surgeon must meticulously attach all of the arteries, veins, and ducts of the organ to the host body. This is the reason the transplant surgeon likes to procure the organ, so as to see the connections in the donor body.

Obviously, transplant surgery is different for each candidate. Each organ is different, the donor is unique, and each candidate and his or her own body is different in its condition and capacity to receive the new organ. In my case, my diseased liver didn't want to leave my body. I was told that much of the surgical time was spent extracting the old liver. I was on the table for ten hours.

A liver transplant, the most difficult of all the transplants, now may take only from four to six hours. Heart and even heart-and-lung transplants generally take even less time. Naturally, the shorter the time one is under anesthesia and receiving blood products, the better and faster one's post-transplant recovery may go. Kidney transplants are the most common, and generally the most easily performed.

Into the ICU

You will usually wake up after your organ transplant in the intensive care unit—in some hospitals, this unit is abbreviated SICU, for Surgical Intensive Care Unit. Often kidney recipients go directly to recovery, but others spend at least one night in the ICU for close monitoring. Having an idea of what to expect will help you face this time with greater ease.

New recipients remain intubated (that is, a breathing tube is inserted into the mouth and extends into the lungs to facilitate breathing) until they are able to breathe on their own, can swallow, and are awake enough to prevent their tongues from blocking their airways. You will be restrained to prevent your pulling out any essential lines while you drift in and out of sleep for a while. You will have several intravenous lines infusing blood and blood products, electrolyte solutions, and intermittent antibiotics into your body. You will also have drains in and around the incision to keep the fluid draining from the space around the transplanted organ, in order to prevent infection.

You will have tight, white nylon support hose on your legs to prevent blood clots. They may be irritating because they are very warm and sometimes cause the skin to itch. There will be tape with a sensor monitor in it around a finger or toe or ear lobe. It registers the amount of oxygen circulating in the blood, so it must be in a vascular place. It has a wire that attaches to a machine, usually over your head, out of sight. It has a red light also, so if it is placed on your finger, you will resemble ET! Some find this line annoying because the wire tugs on the hand in motion.

Recipients often complain about the restraints that are used. Janet explains that they are necessary because the patient has been under anesthesia and has a lot of changes going on in the body. And when the patient wakes up, he or she may be disoriented and confused. The team doesn't know if the first thing someone might do is reach up and pull on the endotracheal tube, which is keeping the recipient ventilated, or pull on a line that supplies vital nutrients. The arms are loosely restrained until the new recipient is extubated or is at least cognitive enough to know what is happening to him or her.

Janet recalls that her husband, David, was confused for several days after his transplant. Janet was with him all the time and, being a nurse, she was sure that she could control what he tugged on and what he didn't.

I had the nurses untie him. He wanted to be able to move his hands. (When someone can't talk, he or she usually tries to talk with his hands.) I felt that I could watch him. I knew what to watch for. I thought that I could accommodate him, giving him a little control. Little did I know that while his hands were untied, under the covers, he was picking at his bypass incision in his groin. He pulled the stitches away, and the incision became infected. He now, seven years later, has a bad scar. I could have prevented that, I knew better.

After years of working with transplant candidates and recipients, there has never been a time when I approach a bedside in the ICU and didn't think of Gulliver awakening to find himself restrained by the thousands of tiny threads tied by the Lilliputians.

This post-transplant sight in the ICU affects all who view it. I did not want my elderly parents to visit me until some of the paraphernalia was gone. Loved ones should understand that you would like them to wait until you feel the situation is more manageable for them.

The length of stay in the ICU depends on the individual and the procedure: the larger the organ, the longer the procedure and the ICU stay, is the general rule. Some might stay two or three days or two to three weeks, depending on their progress. Going in, the new recipient should recognize that the progress is individual; there is no competition. The person who was transplanted before you may be out of intensive care in two or three days, but you don't have to beat that record.

While in the ICU—and throughout your post-transplant recovery—do whatever is asked of you by your medical caregivers, no matter how much you dread it. Get up; sit in a chair. These orders call for mind control; let your mind control your body. Overcome pain and fear. Keep telling yourself that you can do it, whatever "it" is! If you determined before transplant that you were going to be well, then your immediate reaction post-transplant is the proof of your determination. You have two directions before you: to remain weak and indeterminate or to exercise your will power.

Begin moving around. Walk as soon as you possibly can. It is possible that you will have very little pain because many of the nerves that transmit pain were probably cut. It takes several years for the nerves to regenerate. Six years past surgery now, the surface of a part of my abdomen is still numb. If I can pat my head and rub my tummy at the same time, I don't know it!

You will probably have at your disposal a painkiller, a self-dispensing device of morphine or other narcotic. I was told that I used very little of it and really I don't remember much real pain. We are all different this way: some have greater tolerance for pain than others do.

Possible Difficulties and Complications Following Transplant

Usually on the third to about the fifth day post-transplant, a point comes when you feel you have taken a step backward. The day before you felt well, and now you don't. You are a little depressed. In reality, most of the problems that you may face are normal troubles that are probably caused by medication you are taking to prevent your body from rejecting your new organ. Some problems, however, are complications of the surgery, and you should watch out for these.

EMOTION EXTREMES

Massive doses of steroids, given during surgery to trick your immune system into accepting the new organ, can cause extreme emotions. These episodes may manifest in periods of excessive euphoria and exhilaration or other extreme of depression and dejection. Janet and I both remember a woman, just returning to the ward post-transplant, who was having a party, with her confused and tentative husband and a few amused nurses in attendance. She imagined that she had won the lottery and was celebrating amid laughter and chatter. Then there was the patient so depressed post-transplant that she actually died as a result of her resistance to movement. She would not get out of bed, and she would not eat. She became profoundly depressed and would do nothing to help herself or let others help her. Generally, depression this severe is treatable with medication.

Generally patients' moods fall in between these two extremes, and most patients will suffer mild depression toward the end of the first week. Be on the alert for this transient period and use the coping skills you have developed. If you feel like crying, then cry. Don't hold it back because you are afraid it will be perceived as weakness or as a sign that you are giving up. Your transplant team has seen this reaction before.

Janet remembers David having terrible mood swings for a week or two after his transplant. He cried because his favorite baseball team, the Houston Astros, lost a game! It is important to know that you will experience these surges of emotion and to remember that they are caused by steroids—not by lunacy. Your emotions will calm as the steroid doses are reduced and as time passes.

The family needs to prepare for these emotional changes, too. If your newly transplanted relative is depressed, don't panic. It is not a sign of complication or any pathological element. Janet says:

The first time David cried after his transplant was the first time I had ever seen him cry in all the years of our being together. It was devastating to me. I didn't know what I could do to help him. In fact, all I needed to do was understand him and let him express his feelings. I learned to do that. We learned together about the tribulations of being on large amounts of steroids post-transplant and of the Astros having a losing season.

ASCITES

Ascites is the accumulation of fluid in the space between the two layers of membrane that line the abdominal wall. This is a common manifestation of organ failure, particularly liver failure. After transplant, the fluid may leak from the incision site. The leakage is in direct proportion to the fluid accumulation and can be eliminated by diuretics over time. This leakage is most typical in liver transplant recipients. I had a really bad case of it; enough fluid once squirted from my incision site onto a nurse about three feet away that she had to change her scrubs! Most organ recipients probably will not have this problem. Usually the transplant surgeon will put in enough sutures to close the wound. Tubes will be placed to eliminate excessive amounts of drainage.

YOUR BODY'S REJECTION OF THE ORGAN

Your body's immune system is constantly on guard against foreign invaders that may cause it harm. It attacks anything it deems foreign. Most likely, your immune system will not regard your new organ as being part of you (since it really wasn't until just a moment ago) and will attack the organ. This is called rejection of the organ. *Rejection* is a word you will hear often after your transplant. If it occurs, it means that your immune system is winning the war against your new organ. You are not to worry, however. Your transplant team can handle the crisis by increasing or changing your immunosuppressant dosages.

Rejection may cause such symptoms as unexplained fever, flulike symptoms, jaundice, chills, joint and muscle aches, and pain over the transplanted organ. If you experience any of these, call your doctor right away. Sometimes there are no symptoms but doctors detect changes in the results of blood tests. The anticipation of rejection is the primary reason for the constant blood tests that become a routine in the recipient's life.

Lori, another member of the on-line support group for transplant recipients, writes:

> I had a liver rejection six days from transplant. I really didn't feel much different, of course it was early on in the game, but they [the team] could tell because my liver enzymes were elevated, and they performed a biopsy. I received 1,000 milligrams of prednisone every other day during a five-day period. That turned the rejection

around, and now I am twenty-seven months out and have had no other rejection.

Fortunately, I never experienced rejection. On one or two occasions, my liver enzyme levels climbed higher than is desirable, so my medication levels were adjusted in response. I did have an infection in the hospital before discharge. My going home was postponed because of it. I had to begin a ten-day regimen of antibiotics. I left the hospital three weeks after transplant in time for Thanksgiving (was it ever!) at home and did not have to return.

INFECTION

As previously mentioned, after transplant, your immune system will be suppressed in order to prevent it from rejecting your new organ. Of course, there are possible complications that may result. Immunosuppressed patients are much more susceptible to infection—a situation that could be dangerous. Prevention is the best course of action. For these reasons, every effort is made to keep immunosuppressed transplant patients from coming in contact with infectious organisms. The air in the patient's room is usually filtered. Medical staff members don surgical masks and wash their hands before entering transplant patient's rooms. Relatives visiting the patients are required to take the same precautions.

Even after you leave the hospital, you should avoid close contact with people who have contagious diseases. Measles, mumps, and chicken pox are especially dangerous to immunosuppressed persons. If you are exposed to any of these illnesses, notify the transplant coordinator immediately. Remember, good hand-washing is one of the best ways to prevent the transmission and spread of disease.

Hospital Stay on the Ward

When you are recovered enough to be moved from the ICU to a regular hospital ward, which, depending on your rate of recovery could take anywhere from 24 hours to a week or more, your more active role begins. You should get up and start walking as soon as possible. Walking will help increase your circulation, restore your strength, and prevent fluid from accumulating in your lungs. When you begin to walk, you will realize the benefits of walking and exercising before transplant. You will find, amazingly, that you are ready to go again! Janet says to look around and chart a plan; set goals, for example, "Today I will walk to the nurses' station" or "Today I will walk to the elevators."

As time passes and you gain strength, you will begin to focus on going home. It is good to start thinking this way, but the team will decide when you are ready to go home. Some patience is in order. You will probably even feel better immediately after transplant than you have for a long time. As your hopes rise, it may happen that the team arrives for the morning rounds with lab test results that indicate that there may be a problem. The results of any of your routine blood tests may be off. Your "numbers" may be high, they may discover that the incision is not healing just right, or you may have a slight fever, and discharge is postponed. Such postponement is discouraging. You may be inclined to feel that you are regressing. The family may be discouraged too. Nevertheless, it is better to wait a bit for discharge when all is well than to go home too soon and have to return.

David went home three weeks after surgery and should not have. He was back in the hospital in twenty-four hours with a fever. So muster up all the patience you have and understand that your attending hospital staff is doing what's best to restore your health. And be optimistic; many hospital stays are much shorter now due to advanced techniques and the willingness of transplant teams to "let their people go," as they increasingly realize the healing effects of home.

Conclusion

We end Part Two on an optimistic note. Finally there is an organ match, after an intense and anxious wait. You receive a call to come to the hospital in response to someone else's generous gift. Your life will be extended, and that gift will keep on giving. The transplant surgery lasts from six to ten hours or more, depending on the condition of the organ and the recipient. The ICU and hospital ward stay are also variable, but the one certainty is that you will go home feeling healthier, stronger, and more forward-looking than you have in a very long time.

Let's explore your life outside the hospital now after your transplant.

PART THREE

Post-Transplant

CHAPTER SEVEN

Compliance with Medications and Other Post-Transplant Care

Unlike the preceding chapters, this chapter discusses not temporary, passing issues that are irrelevant once you recover, but issues that will be relevant for the rest of your life. Unless there is some major scientific advance in the field of transplantation in the near future, you will be on immunosuppressant medication from the time of surgery on. The good news is that you will be most immunosuppressed during the days following the transplant in the hospital. Thereafter, once you are stabilized, your dosages will be reduced.

You will find, upon discharge, that your life revolves around a medication regimen. Janet says that this constant preoccupation is good because you will assume the habits that will support you in future compliance. That future compliance depends in part on your understanding of the role of prescribed medications in your transplant recovery and in your post-transplant health. We discuss those medications in this chapter. (When we present a medication, we will first use the brand name that professionals are more likely to use and then the generic name, which is more common when professionals speak to patients. The generic name is presented in parentheses. Along the way we will drop the brand names and use the generic name, which you will hear used more often.)

Before we explore the limitless combinations of medication, I want to address you, the patient, as I do with my patients face to face, about the use of generic drugs. Transplant is a relatively new phenomenon and has brought with it new drugs often spoken of as cutting-edge immunosuppressive therapies. Until recently, brand-name drugs were the only ones of their kind in this market of what is considered critical dose drugs (those for which maintaining appropriate blood levels is critical to the action of the drug). Some of these drugs have lost their patent and have given other major pharmaceutical companies the opportunity to develop new formulations of that drug and market it as such under a new name by a new company. Such is the case with cyclosporine A (the generic name). It is currently available in three formulations: Neoral by Novartis, Gengraf by Abbott, and Eon by Eon Laboratories. The latter two modified formulations have been tested by the Food and Drug Administration (FDA) and considered bioequivalent to the Neoral made by Novartis Pharmaceuticals. The big debate in the bioequivalent arena is that FDA testing is not performed in a manner that yields a true equal test. This scenario is, and probably always will be, debatable with any modified formulations of brand-name drugs, not just immunosuppressants. This testing and the data that is examined in transplant centers across the United States is not for you, the patient, to be concerned about. Your transplant team has too much already invested in your improved quality of life to allow substituting a drug that will not benefit your newly transplanted organ. The more realistic debate is whether the pharmacy chain or third-party pay (or your insurance carrier) can dictate switching of a brand-named, critical-dosed drug to a generic-critical dosed drug without notifying or receiving permission from the transplant team to do so. Unfortunately, it is common practice when it comes to antibiotics, diuretics, and numerous other medications you receive today. If you don't believe me, think back to the last two times you were given an antibiotic prescription and had it filled at your local pharmacy. Did the tablets or capsules look the same? Chances are great that they did not! A generic brand was substituted for the brand prescribed for you by your physician, who neglected to mark the required box specifying "Do not substitute" or "Dispense as written." With drugs other than critical-dose medications, chances are that they are OK and do the job your physician intended them to do. No harm was done because your team of medical professionals did not get the message regarding the substitution. However, with drugs such as cyclosporine A it does matter that we know. Consistency is the name of the game when dealing with critical-dose drugs. Whether it is consistency with regards to times, dosage, or formulation, we like consistency.

Immunosuppressants

Simply put, your immune system is designed to attack foreign materials. That attack mechanism means that bacteria and viruses can be identified and destroyed before they can injure your body. In the person with a transplanted organ, those front-line warriors of the immune system do not recognize the foreign organ as anything but an enemy, a foreign body to be destroyed.

Your team has access to a variety of medications for avoiding organ rejection. The first to make transplant survival possible back in the early 1980s was cyclosporine. Other immunosuppressants include Gengraf, Prograf, Eon, CellCept, Imuran, Rapammune, and prednisone. Your transplant team will use a combination of two or three of these drugs. A combination is useful because they all have slightly different methods of action and because the recipient is spared the side effects resulting from a large dose of one drug. They all have side effects. We will explain these and how to cope with them later on.

You will be as immune suppressed as you will ever be immediately after transplant and the first three to six months thereafter. The team will watch you closely for any signs of infection, which is always a risk in a hospital setting. Because you are immune suppressed, you are vulnerable to infection. The good news is that the farther you are from transplant, the less immune suppressed you will be and the more you may tolerate exposures to a common cold, for example.

Immunosuppressant medications are necessary to reduce the power of the immune system, thereby protecting the new organ from the immune system's assault. A combination of immunosuppressant drugs is used to prevent rejection of the new organ.

Despite the fact that many experts express differing strong opinions about what works best and what should be done, almost everyone agrees that the best way to manage immunosuppression is by individualizing treatment. What works for one doesn't always work for another. One patient may experience a side effect while taking a drug, while another won't.

Immunosuppression is currently a two-edged sword. We certainly have the ability to prevent and eliminate rejection, but the drugs have profound side effects, particularly when given intensively, at high doses. All decisions have to be made by weighing the risk versus the benefit. Such decisions are difficult when risks and benefits are not completely determined. Much progress has been made, but we still have a long way to go.

CYCLOSPORINE

Until the introduction of cyclosporine in the early 1980s, a much larger percentage of transplants failed because of rejection. Your doctor may prescribe cyclosporine under different brand names, including Neoral, Sandimmune, Gengraf, or Eon. This drug inhibits the action of the immune cells called T-lymphocytes. It is the drug of choice particularly for most kidney and heart transplant recipients.

AZATHIOPRINE

Azathioprine (Imuran) may be prescribed as an adjunctive therapy along with cyclosporine. This agent appears to work by altering the DNA of the cells of the immune system, inhibiting antibody production. It is the oldest immunosuppressant, with the exception of steroids.

TACROLIMUS

Tacrolimus (Prograf) works by preventing the action of the T-lymphocytes. It is one of the newer immunosuppressive agents used by the vast majority of liver transplant centers.

MYCOPHENOLATE MOFETIL

Some centers administer mycophenolate mofetil (CellCept) immediately after transplant to prevent rejection; others use it as a "rescue therapy," that is, to treat acute rejection episodes. Janet says of her center: "If a recipient has an acute rejection episode within two or three months post-transplant, then we admit the person and administer steroids and CellCept. In six months to a year, almost all centers discontinue Cell-Cept."

PREDNISONE

Prednisone is used as an immunosuppressant in conjunction with one of the agents already mentioned. It is dispensed under several brand names. It is a steroid, which produces undesirable side effects, including bone loss, when used over a long period of time. Most transplant teams begin to wean the recipient from prednisone relatively early after transplant. Heart recipients remain on prednisone longer than other solid organ recipients do. Each center has its own protocol.

SIDE EFFECTS OF IMMUNOSUPPRESSIVE MEDICATIONS

While transplant would not be possible without immunosuppressant agents, these drugs' benefits do not come without costs. Immunosuppressants cause side effects that range in severity from troublesome to life-threatening.

Some common side effects of immunosuppressants include hypertension, hair loss, excessive hair growth, tremors, edema (swelling due to accumulation of fluid), excessive bruising, headaches, hyperlipidemia (high blood cholesterol and triglyceride levels), acne, gum disease, gastrointestinal distress, osteoporosis, infection, weight gain, and skin cancer.

Some precautions can be taken against these side effects: Exercise regularly and eliminate some of the risk factors for hypertension and hyperlipidemia, such as obesity; a high-fat, high-cholesterol diet; smoking; and a high salt intake. Follow a low-fat diet that emphasizes fruits and vegetables and contains lots of potassium, calcium, and magnesium and minimizes salt and sugar. This will help minimize the risk of hypertension, hyperlipidemia, and edema. Regularly monitor blood level and blood pressure changes. Condition your hair regularly to minimize breakage. Also avoid hair-damaging processes, such as perming, dyeing, and bleaching and limit your exposure to chlorine and the sun. Maintain good dental hygiene and avoid smoking to limit gum disease. See your dentist at least twice a year.

Some more serious side effects to watch out for are bloody or black stools, irregular heartbeat, fever, chills, seizures, convulsions, shortness of breath, confusion, and numbness in the hands or feet. Notify your doctor right away if you experience any of these symptoms. There are studies that imply that tacrolimus may produce more neurological side effects than cyclosporine. There may be some central nervous system disorders with symptoms such as tingling in the extremities or blurred vision.

Janet suggests that these side effects may be used as diagnostic tools. There is an ideal level of immunosuppressant drugs in the body's system. If you note that your headaches are more intense than usual or that you are experiencing tremors, then you should assume that the medications are at a toxic level, and a call to the coordinator may be in order. Often this assumption is correct, and the physician will adjust the dosage accordingly.

Janet and I remember a recipient, Charles, who would call to say that he couldn't keep his noodles in his spoon. This alert meant that his hand shook when he tried to eat chicken noodle soup, which was a part of his daily lunch. The complaint became a kind of code for Charles and Janet. If he couldn't keep his noodles in his spoon, his cyclosporine level was usually too high. More often than not, subsequent blood tests indicated that an adjustment was in order. Whatever works! Many recipients get so in tune with their bodies that they can come close to predicting their blood levels, just as a lifelong diabetic can usually tell a physician what his or her blood sugar level is at any given time of the day. When tested, sure enough, they are usually within ten points one way or the other.

For myself, in the first year after transplant, the unpleasant side effects of cyclosporine were neuropathy in my feet and insomnia. When both of these signs were acute and worsened, I called Janet. More often than not, my cyclosporine dosage was lowered. After the introduction of tacrolimus, also known as FK506, many recipients were switched from cyclosporine to tacrolimus if they were experiencing troublesome side effects. I was not, simply because the side effect that often accompanied cyclosporine was neural in nature, and I already had enough neuropathy, thank you. Switching might have intensified my symptoms. The transplant team will introduce the medication most suited to the individual recipient.

Finally, do not take cyclosporine or tacrolimus with grapefruit juice or drink any for an hour after dosage. Studies show that grapefruit juice increases the blood levels of cyclosporine and tacrolimus. Orange juice and other juices are fine.

Other Prophylactic Post-Transplant Medications

Preemptive or prophylactic medications are those taken to prevent a medical problem. Because of the significant amount of immunosuppression immediately following transplant and the high degree of susceptibility to infection for the first year following transplant, recipients may be required to take some of the following:

AN ANTIBACTERIAL AGENT

An example of an antibacterial agent is (SMZ/TMP) Bactrim, which is a prophylactic against pneumocystic pneumonia.

AN ANTIVIRAL AGENT

Ganciclovir sodium (Cytovene) and amantadine hydrochloride (Symmetrel) are examples of antiviral agents. Amantadine is believed to be an effective agent to reduce the viral load in recipients who have hepatitis C. Like any drug, however, it is not without side effects, and its use in this capacity is still controversial.

ANTIFUNGAL MEDICATIONS

These medications are used to counteract fungal illnesses such as candidiasis and cryptococcal meningitis. Nystatin (Mycostatin) mouth rinse and pastilles can prevent oral thrush.

DIURETICS

Diuretics such as furosemide (Lasix) may be used to ease the water retention that commonly follows transplant. Diuretics are used in moderation for the post-transplant patient to reduce swelling in extremities and to reduce the amount of ascites in the abdomen and correct fluid overload. This medication works also to regulate blood pressure.

ANTIHYPERTENSIVE MEDICATIONS

These drugs are used for those recipients with high blood pressure, which is sometimes a side effect of immunosuppressant drugs. An antihypertensive may be needed immediately after transplant, but not over time. The body must adjust after surgery; it is retaining fluid, but after a time, the hypertensive drug will probably be withdrawn.

AN ANTIULCER AGENT

This medication prevents gastric irritation resulting from steroid therapy.

MAGNESIUM OXIDE

Magnesium oxide is a replacement therapy for the body's loss of magnesium due to immunosuppressant agents. Most immunosuppressive medications work by binding to different minerals circulating in the blood. Magnesium is the mineral most affected by this mechanism. This reaction causes the magnesium usually circulating in your blood to be excreted in urine. Over-the-counter drugs are just as good as prescription drugs and are cheaper.

PRAVASTATIN SODIUM

Pravastatin sodium (Pravachol) reduces blood lipid (fat) levels. This medication is prescribed for those recipients with elevated cholesterol and triglycerides. Current studies reveal that pravastatin may also have some immunosuppressive action in post-transplant patients.

UROSODIOL

Urosodiol (Actigall, Urso) is a bile acid used to thin bile and prevent cholestasis in the liver. Cholestasis is an obstruction of the flow of bile. This medication is important for liver recipients.

Adjusting and Scheduling Medication Post-Transplant

Remember that you will be on the highest dose of antirejection drugs when you are discharged than at any other time. By six months after transplant, and certainly by one year, you will be taking far less medication. Generally, six months after discharge you will be taking one-half the original dosage, and by one year out, half again of that.

The more the recipient eats and exercises, the more the levels of immunosuppressants need adjusting. These agents work to suppress the immune system of the recipient for a twelve-hour cycle. The medications, in order to prevent rejection of the transplanted organ, must be taken every twelve hours. Usually the recipient chooses the times most convenient for his or her lifestyle; for example, 8 a.m. and 8 p.m., 9 a.m. and 9 p.m., or 5 a.m. and 5 p.m. You will be asked to decide before you leave the hospital on a time best suited to your lifestyle for taking medications. These times are not necessarily written in stone, but once you choose the times, stick to your plan. The purpose is to keep the level of the immunosuppressant drug in the bloodstream constant in order to achieve its maximum effect as an antirejection agent. Consider your lifestyle before choosing the times. You might, for example, like to stay up late at night and then sleep late the next day, or vice versa. The team regularly monitors your blood level of the drugs through blood tests. Based on the blood test results, they may increase or decrease the dosage.

Janet recalls a pediatric recipient who didn't want to go to kindergarten because when the nurse came into the classroom promptly at 8 a.m. with her morning meds, the other kids made fun of her. One phone call to the coordinator took care of this sensitive matter. The mother had not understood that the regimen followed in the hospital was not written in stone. She made a simple hour adjustment to 7 a.m. and 7 p.m., and all was well. The little girl could take her medication at home before leaving for school.

Another recipient told Janet once that he could not tolerate his immunosuppression medications when he took them with his other morning medications. Every time he tried, he would get nauseated and throw up. Nothing seemed to help until one day Janet discovered that he was taking his Bactrim, an antibiotic, every morning. Often this medication can cause some gastrointestinal discomfort. Janet has found that taking it at bedtime is the better option. Once he made that minor adjustment, he was fine.

Medication and the Need for Communication

Here we repeat the admonition: *Never take any medication, prescribed by another physician or over the counter, without consulting your transplant team* (and be sure to notify any doctor or dentist you see of the medications you are taking).

Remember also that while herbal remedies may be fine for most, transplant patients must use caution. Even cold lozenges with zinc, for example, or the popular Saint John's wort should not be taken without consultation. Many drugs and herbal remedies on the market can cause a rejection episode or a high toxic level when interacting with your other medications. Herbal remedies may not come to mind when the transplant team asks you if you have taken any medication the team has not prescribed. Many do not consider these types of home remedies to be medication. Keep in mind that even the slightest indiscretion may alter your immunosuppression level enough to cause problems.

The transplant recipient is encouraged to call the transplant team for any valid reason. The candidate and his or her family receive extensive education on side effects, possible drug interactions, and signs and symptoms of infection. These classes are given frequently, and the teaching is reinforced throughout the wait time, in-house prior to discharge, at support group meetings, and in clinic follow-up visits.

If you miss a dose of medication by four hours or more, you should call the transplant coordinator for instructions. If you are less than two hours late in taking your dose, the medication should be taken at discovery. Increasingly, the recipient must be responsible for his or her own wellness. We will address the issue of compliance shortly.

The Pharmacy's Role
in Transplant Medication

You will leave the hospital after transplant with more medication than at any other time in your life. You and your caregiver may be discouraged at the beginning. The entire medication routine may seem overwhelming. The caregiver will hesitate to leave the new recipient, still weak from surgery, to go out to the pharmacy and will be especially frustrated if the ordered medication has not yet arrived.

Janet suggests that you or your caregiver research the pharmaceutical service early in the pre-transplant period, as we mentioned earlier. Find a pharmacist with whom you can talk, explain what medications you will be on, and work out a plan. Then when the support person goes to the pharmacist upon your discharge, your needs will be met. Your medications will be changed a lot at first, as we said, so you and your pharmacist will become well acquainted.

Some centers may refer you to a pharmacy that is experienced in serving transplant recipients. For most transplant recipients that pharmacy will not be local, but there will be an 800 number always available for distant service. I have used one, and I have been amazed at how quickly the medications were mailed to me, even overnight without extra charge. Working with such a pharmacy can be an advantage. It may supply you with a package of necessary items upon discharge, such as a blood pressure cuff, a thermometer, a pill cutter, and a weekly pillbox. The nurse educator may send you home with a month's supply of medicine from this pharmacy.

These transplant pharmacies are a coordinator's security blanket. They may notify the recipient if they have not received renewals in the appropriate time. They sometimes have full-time financial coordinators and social workers. The recipient can speak directly with the pharmacist who filled his or her prescriptions. He knows what he is talking about; your local drugstore pharmacist may not be as familiar with some of the immunosuppressive agents.

Speaking of refills, make sure you stay on top of the amount of medication you have left. Don't call your coordinator on Friday at 5 p.m. and tell her you've just taken your last pill. Keep track of your medications and recognize the need to call for refills ahead of time, keeping in mind that if you are using a mail-order or specialty pharmacy, a week is not long enough for the refill.

Travel and Your Medication

If you are traveling outside the country, you should ask the center for a letter that lists the medications you are taking as a transplant recipient. You do not want to end up in jail. You may need the affidavit for customs. Keep your medications in the prescription bottle with the pharmacy label in which they came. Many countries require the pharmacy-dispensing label to confirm the contents. Be sure to take more medication than you will need; you never know what circumstance may delay your returning home. In fact, if you commute some distance to work, it would be good to keep one or two doses, especially of immunosuppressive medication, on your person or in your purse or briefcase. These drugs should be kept at room temperature and in their containers, so leaving them in the car is not an option.

If you are traveling by air, always take all of your medication with you in a carry-on bag. We've all heard stories about lost luggage. If you are checking your luggage on a flight or train, don't pack your medication. You may never see it again! The last thing you want to have happen is to arrive at your destination with no clothes *and* no medication. You can find a place to buy clothes; but imagine trying to find a place to buy immuno-suppression medications!

Nutrition

Adequate calories and protein are important for healing after surgery. Structure your diet plan so that it allows you to meet your needs as well as maintain a good weight for you. It is important to include a variety of foods, particularly fruits and vegetables, in your nutrition program. It is wise to be moderate in using fats and sugars. This vigilance will promote good health and control your weight.

The typical transplant recipient does not want to eat much after surgery. He or she just has little appetite. The team or the primary care-giver has to urge the recipient to eat. And then, later . . . watch out for the prednisone munchies! You may find yourself eating the kitchen table. This is when you had better walk or do some other exercise to maintain your weight! David used to call it the forced march. I looked rather svelte after transplant and thought I could eat with impunity. Wrong! Six years later I am still trying to get back to what I looked like at discharge.

Conclusion

The information in this chapter may give you the impression that you will be spending every waking hour just attending to your newly transplanted self. One good thing about us humans is that we assume habits and adapt rather easily. In fact, that adaptation is how we got this high on the evolutionary totem pole. Some of the regimens, especially with regard to medication, will be reduced or eliminated as you move away from the surgery. The remaining procedures and recommendations will become second nature. You will be compliant most of the time without much thought. The areas where you tend to be forgetful will be the ones that will need your attention. Just keep in mind what it is that you have to take care of—a fellow human's living gift, and your own precious health.

CHAPTER EIGHT

Coping with Post-Transplant Emotions

After leaving the hospital and upon returning home you are likely to experience a rush of emotions. There are sound reasons for emotional reactions, even conflicting ones. You have been through the stress of surgery after the stress of waiting, and you have come through successfully. Now you face the future with a degree of uncertainty. You may feel uncertain about your self, your identity, your body, and your future. And don't forget about the large doses of prednisone you've been taking. This medication enhances emotion, whether emotional highs or lows, and affects different people differently.

In this chapter, we discuss your range of emotions and conflicts, as well as your body image and other relevant matters of identity, including your feelings toward your donor. We will discuss, in a way, the remainder of your life as a transplant recipient. This post-transplant time is a good time, but it is not without its concerns and problems.

Separation Anxiety/Dependence

A new recipient is often torn between dependence and independence. You have been exercising a great deal of dependence throughout your illness. Most of what you have learned from your team and from this book emphasizes your following some very definite restrictions and recommendations. The consequences could be dire should you deviate from instructions. You have formed attitudes and habits of dependence. Whatever temperament is naturally yours—perhaps to be radically independent—you have had to suppress in order to be compliant and to get well. Obviously there are two opposite behaviors that, in the extreme, are dangerous for the recipient. You might be totally dependent on the team or on your support person, or you might choose to return to your pre-transplant life, ignoring new necessary and helpful behaviors.

Every recipient hesitates a little and is a bit reluctant at the thought of discharge. The team has been on the receiving end of the buzzer during any and every hospital stay. They will still be at the other end of a telephone call, but you may be some distance away. Anxiety over your ability to keep up with medication and other practices is natural. You may have the "what ifs" uppermost in your mind. Most recipients will find the stable place between anxiety and complacency.

The truly professional transplant team will begin weaning the recipient from total dependence even in the surgical ICU. The recipient, in turn, will practice internalizing his or her regimen so that it really becomes his or her own. You will assume responsibility for your wellness even as you continue to have assistance along the way.

Janet has observed that older recipients tend to have more of a problem with the post-transplant period. They don't move around as much as they should in order to gain strength, and they have a difficult time separating from the transplant team at the time of discharge. Janet says:

We are treating a woman at this time who had a difficult post-op period. Consequently, she was in and out of the hospital several times post-transplant. She has become very dependent on us and on her husband, who had quit work at the time to be with her. Now that she is doing well, he has gone back to work. She calls our office now with little complaints periodically and ends up having to come to the ER. We find that when she gets there, she's fine. It is as if it is therapeutic treatment to come to the ER and see us and be reassured that she's OK.

Let's face it, the easiest course of action for the transplant team is to have the candidate be totally obedient to their orders before transplant and totally independent after discharge, while, of course, being compliant and having no complications. This scenario has never existed. The team must be patient while the recipient increasingly takes charge of his or her own health. Regular clinic visits will come to replace frantic calls in the night and ER visits. These clinic visits will become fewer and fewer and will finally occur only when the team is adjusting medications or if there is a problem.

Some recipients, especially men, turn their wellness care over to their spouses. Some others continue to depend too much on their support persons. The matter may be simply habit manifesting itself. In the family, it is the wife/mother who tends to the family's health needs more often than not. She makes dental and doctor appointments, monitors checkups, orders prescriptions from the pharmacist, and nurses as she nurtures her family. These matters often are not in the husband's realm. Clearly an adjustment is in order.

I remember some remarks from wives of recipients in my support group. One spoke of her husband sleeping late on weekends and how she woke him to take his medicine on time. Another stated that her husband did not know the correct dosages of his medications, he had turned everything over to her. The scary thing is that she adjusted his medication according to what she perceived about his side effects!

Let me mention here another trait that I noticed among some recipient couples. Sometimes it appears that a spouse has finally achieved the degree of control that he or she has wanted. The recipient is dependent on her and grateful. The caregiver is happy to keep him that way. Obviously this is not good for the recipient. It is his or her responsibility to stay well.

Dependence of this kind reveals a passive attitude toward any post-transplant obstacles.

Fear of Rejection of the Organ

Fear of transplant rejection is a completely rational fear. It is a possible complication of the procedure, and it could be life-threatening. It certainly doesn't help matters, however, to live the rest of your life in fear of such an event. Try to remember that the statistics are with you. The vast majority of transplants are successful, and recipients go on to live normal, productive lives. Also remember that if your body does begin to reject your transplanted organ, all is not lost. Doctors can make adjustments to stop rejection. Just remember to take your medications religiously, and follow all of the guidelines that your transplant team gives you. Try some of the relaxation techniques outlined in chapter 4 to help ease your fears. As time goes on, your fears will abate, especially if you never experience rejection.

Euphoria

Most transplant recipients, even in the midst of feelings of temerity, feel euphoric after transplant, especially upon returning home. That just may be the best high a human being can experience. It is a wonderful sensation. The emotion is understood as a feeling of well-being, relaxation, and happiness. I felt whole again, on a sure path to health, to being able to feel well again. Most transplant recipients have not believed that wellness could be a part of their lives for a very long time. There is now a future, and it feels great! People who have been sick for a long time lose their optimism.

To the extent that one has been stressed, one now feels proportionately relaxed. We have found that the transplant procedure from diagnosis to discharge is one prolonged, unrelieved stressor. That has been replaced by exuberance and well-being.

A medical anthropologist, Leslie Sharp, interviewed a number of recipients who expressed a sense of having been reborn or having a new lease on life:

> *Many of my informants also celebrate the day of their transplant as a second birthday or "rebirthday" (complete with a cake shaped like the organ). When recipients receive the call from the hospital informing them that a matching organ has been found, the scene that ensues at home is most often compared to a young couple setting off for the birth of their first child. The recipient is compared to an expectant mother who waits patiently as her spouse or other kin rush about in a panic, searching frantically for the prepacked suitcase, and then struggle clumsily in their attempts to start the car.*

This quotation aptly summarizes my actions upon receiving the call.

In my support group, it was a tradition, if one can call a few years' practice a tradition, to celebrate the first anniversary of transplant with a cake shared by all and a gift to the recipient. The gift was always a T-shirt with the date of the person's transplant on it. I used my own first-year anniversary to thank all those who had supported me in a close and personal way through my transplant. We had a big party at my expense. Yes, David and Janet were there.

Guilt

Many of us do not know what to do with a gift. We even have to practice saying what we will say upon accepting one. We are uncomfortable. Feelings of guilt often arise post-transplant. Almost every recipient goes through a guilt phase. Some feel a survivor's guilt. They may be preoccupied with the thought that someone else had to die for them to live, or they may feel guilty because some others did not live to undergo transplant. Remember that these feelings are just that—feelings. These guilty feelings result from incorrect logic, from unclear thinking. A transplant recipient, as we have said, is not alive *because* someone died but because someone wanted to be an organ donor. The recipient had absolutely nothing to do with the donor's death. The recipient's living is the result of the generosity of another. It may be that this generosity is a difficult concept to grasp. The fact that you received a transplant and someone else did not is also beyond your control. It may even be that your success had something to do with your efforts, the kind we discussed in Part One. For that, you should be congratulated. You must forgive yourself and love yourself and thereby turn outward and reciprocate in the best way you can. We will have more to say later about reciprocation, a felt need of every transplant recipient.

Jim Gleason, a heart recipient, who is almost always present in transplant forums, sent a little ditty to the on-line group. He did not identify its origin. I quote from a part of it here:

> *One thing kept going through my mind. I can't change yesterday, but I do have the power to make today a wonderful day. I can be happy, joyous, fulfilled, encouraged, as well as encouraging. Knowing this, I left the City of Regret immediately and left no forwarding address. Am I sorry for mistakes I've made in the past? Yes! But there is no physical way to undo them. So, if you're planning a trip back to the City of Regret, please cancel all of your reservations now. Instead, take a trip to a place called Starting Again. I liked it so much that I have now taken up permanent residence there. My neighbors, the I Forgive Myselfs and the New Starts, are so very helpful. By the way, you don't have to carry around heavy baggage, because the load is lifted from your shoulders upon arrival. If you can find this great town—it is in your own heart—please look me up. I live on I Can Do It Street.*

Jim is known in transplant circles as the "Cookie Monster" because he is so upbeat, like the Sesame Street character. Like most people who love themselves and others, he has done exceedingly well post-transplant. Look him up, especially if you are a fiftyish guy with a heart transplant. He has his own website where you can read an account of his book in progress about his own transplant adventure.

Feelings of Victimization

There are those who have experienced the failure of an organ through no fault of their own. If they do not find a place for their experience, they too, like those who feel guilt, can succumb to depression. The feeling of "I don't deserve this suffering" is neither comfortable nor productive. The problem with both sets of feelings is that it is easy to take one's self off the hook of personal responsibility. Instead of getting with the program of wellness and working toward health, as a recipient must, the guilty or the victimized recipient just lives in his or her own self-indulgence.

Peter Whybrow, M.D., says that "self-knowledge is the big key to regaining one's health." Writing about a friend of his who is manic-depressive, he quotes his friend, who is also a psychiatrist: "[Manic] depression is an underworld, a world where it is difficult to learn the truth of things, and where it is dangerous to live. Only in standing back from that realm have I come to recognize that life's true beauty is in its balance and its harmony. I am content now, in the place where I have found myself." While the recipient's feelings may not be as extreme perhaps as manic-depression, one can, nevertheless, find oneself in a negative realm where powerful feelings can assert themselves to no good end. There is a balance and a harmony that one must work to attain, never allowing these negative feelings to prevail.

I think one of the reasons I have such affection for David is that he could have played the victim but he chose not to. As well as he and Janet can understand, David seems to have become infected with hepatitis C while serving as a paramedic with the fire department, before the advent of protective gloves. He was treating an injured person who had the hepatitis C virus. He has chosen not to play the victim's role. Instead, he has retrained since transplant and has become a surgical technician.

Egoism

Transplantation has probably distinguished the recipient among his or her peers. In any one social group, there is not likely to be more than one transplanted member, unless it is a transplant support group! It is very easy for a recipient to become socially obnoxious. Usually this is acted out in a self-promoting way. The recipient gives an "organ recital," talking about the experience anytime he or she can. People will view the recipient as unique, at least for awhile, and ask questions. These questions can easily foster a one-way dissertation that goes on and on.

The recipient is in a position to do a lot of good for the transplant cause, talking up donation and representing success. Unfortunately, one can also reverse one's impact by becoming self-promoting. We all have to guard against this imposition on others. Really, all we have to do is think a little about even what we are called, "recipient." We have been given a gift. Just as with our original gift of life, we have not done anything to merit it.

Don't Forget About Your Caregiver

After all that your caregiver has done for you, you may feel beholden to him or her. The best reward for him or her is probably just getting back to normal. Undoubtedly this person has sacrificed a great deal in order to care for you. He or she has endured significant stress simply out of love for you. You can best thank this person by turning attention away from yourself now and becoming considerate of his or her needs.

For a time after discharge, you may still require care. Someone else may have to drive for you and provide some necessities. It won't be long, though, before you can relieve your caregiver of the added burdens and begin to do for him or her again. Actually, you'll feel great being useful again.

As recipients we have gotten used to being cared for, to having our every need met. We really have to break some of these habits and become self-sufficient again and less preoccupied with ourselves. If your caregiver has stuck with you this long, he or she is probably fed up and ready for a change! This is the person to reach out to first. Do for this person whatever your means and circumstances allow. Just little things, tokens of appreciation, will mean so much. As for you, these little generous acts will begin to move you out of yourself. You have had to focus on yourself in order to get well, but now it is time to turn outward. It is easy to continue the habits of receiving. Obviously, altruism or generosity of spirit is a value promoted in much of this book. The purpose of this emphasis is ultimately therapeutic. Have you ever known a happy, fulfilled selfish person—Not a self-fulfilled person whose life is expansive, but a self-centered person whose life is confined to a very narrow circumference? We cannot continue, for our own sake, to simply take.

If your caregiver is strained, overworked, and exhausted, see to it. The psychiatrist member of the transplant team is available for your support persons too, even for the entire family if that is necessary. A few visits to this transplant team member may be helpful in order for you and your family to get your life back on track. This specialist is available to help you deal with any post-transplant emotional issues, such as those we have discussed. If you feel overwrought with guilt, or if the prednisone is causing you to cry or rage uncontrollably, make an appointment. These matters can be talked through. There is a reason that a psychiatrist or a psychologist is a member of the transplant team. Others before you have faced an emotional chasm too broad to fly over alone.

Post-Transplant Feelings for the Donor

In spite of medical professionals' attempt to depersonalize contributed organs and maintain anonymity and distance, some recipients struggle with various aspects of donor identification.

A GIFT FROM A STRANGER

For those who have difficulty accepting an outright gift of any kind, it may be very difficult to accept such a precious gift from a stranger. Let us consider here very plainly again what happens in organ transplantation. A part of another's body is planted in yours. It becomes yours physically because it is connected to your veins and arteries. It is your blood that gives life to the organ, that allows it to pump or pulse again and to perform vital functions. Now, how do you feel about whose organ it is, and who you are? The body's boundaries have been expanded. Most transplant centers do not provide much information about the organ donor. Some recipients put together what they know and construct their own image of the donor. Sometimes they attempt to integrate this other personality with their own. There are always interesting anecdotes about a recipient's change in dietary habits. Do you feel as though you have, post-transplant, a new sense of self?

Leslie Sharp tells us:

Recipients, as they attempt to define themselves post-transplant, must reflect on how organs affect the functioning of their reconstructed body. Their new self is defined in reference to changes that have occurred in bodies that were at one time fragile and worn from illness. Rebirth is a dominant idiom that recipients use to express their transformation, which they describe as miraculous outcomes borne forth by sophisticated medical technology. From the donor's death springs the revived recipient, who, under any other medical circumstances, would have died.

It may be that if we persist in seeing the donated organ as "other" and its donor as a stranger, and these perceptions trouble us, our problem lies in our view of humanity. We do not think of people as our brothers and sisters in the human race. If we did, it would be natural, not extraordinary, to donate organs and to conserve donated organs with care so that we don't use up another person's chance at life.

I know quite a bit about my donor, but not his name. I could have known that, had I cared to. I still could, I suppose. He died of a head wound in a drive-by shooting in Dallas. He was in the wrong place at the wrong time—an innocent bystander. I could check out the event in a Dallas newspaper. It doesn't seem necessary. The one outstanding feature that has stayed vividly with me is the fact that he was a university student who had learned about organ donation on campus at a lecture he attended. Now that is a coincidence. I teach students about his age on a university campus. I am careful to talk with them about organ donation. Sometimes I think that my donor represented a kind of "thank you" from hundreds of students whom I have tried to influence for the good. I say this quite humbly. You see, then, that I have created a kind of narrative around my donor. I try to pay him back by continuing to attend to university students. I have found a place for his identity in relation to mine. I think most recipients do roughly the same. You will with time find a place for this new unsought relationship.

Janet had encouraged me to write to my donor's family to thank them for their gift to me. She mailed the letter; the donor remained anonymous to me. I expect that she had in mind the bereaved family of my young donor. What the letter did for me, however, was allow me to personalize the donor, to recognize his "otherness." He had a family, a place of origin, a history. I received one of his organs but not his identity. I was I, and he was he.

THE KNOWN DONOR

In spite of everyone's best efforts, the living related or unrelated organ donation can get a bit sticky. According to Sharp, "The ties that bind the living, known donor to the kidney recipient generate a complicated set of emotions that can surpass the love or hatred felt for other family members. Conflicts arise over boundaries that define whose kidney it is, and donors may insist upon their right, as one informant put it, to protect their kidney."

Whose organ is it anyway? In one family everyone except Patricia, the recipient, refers to the transplanted kidney as Billy's, even though it has been housed in her body for half her life. Clearly some understanding must be reached. In these cases, at least the persons involved can talk it out. It may be that a third person counselor can assist. There is certainly nothing wrong with expressions of gratitude. If the donor is demanding, however, some closure is necessary. It might help for the recipient to write a letter to the donor, just as recipients from anonymous, cadaver donors write to the family. Express your gratitude in a heartfelt way and then get on with your life. Transplantation should not take over your life in the sense of its being the be-all and end-all of your every thought and action.

FEELING THE NEED TO RECIPROCATE

Every organ recipient feels anxious to do something in exchange for the priceless gift of life. Most find a way to reciprocate by working as advocates for organ donation. Others extend themselves to new members in their transplant support group.

There really can't be too many advocates for organ donation, considering the scarcity of organ donors. Something about our contemporary society seems to cause people to resist organ donation. The recipient who wants to be active in this sphere can hook up with existing organizations easily. Your own transplant coordinator can put you in touch with a local organization—local for you, that is, should you live some distance from your center.

These organizations and support groups are formed under many different names. Some of them can be found in the back of this book. If none of these appear to be available to you, contact your nearest organ procurement organization (OPO).

Your whole life need not be donated to transplant causes. In fact, none of it *has to* be. You will always be a kind of walking testimony to the success of organ transplantation. You were on the receiving end of a medical marvel in order to get well. That is all that you *must* do. You were healed in order for you to get on with your life. Don't fixate on an agenda as the result of "the tyranny of the gift." A gift comes without strings attached. Again, try to be comfortable with this amazing good fortune. People who win the lottery don't run around saying that they are unworthy. On the other hand, some of them say spontaneously that they will give a percentage of their winnings to charity. Perhaps that is a good analogy for organ winners. In many ways, ours has been the luck of the draw, and it is good to spread the good fortune around.

Conclusion

Sometimes the cluster of post-transplant emotions can be overwhelming. You may experience negative emotions of fear and guilt, as well as positive feelings of gratitude and relief—even euphoria. Any and all feelings are enhanced by the steroid prednisone and will subside as the dose does. There is a place for happiness and for sharing that happiness with those around you. Should emotions overwhelm you, look to the transplant team as you have throughout the process. Your coordinator can give you a list of transplant support groups near your home. These groups are a wonderful resource for exercising your new energies positively, for offering you current information, and for giving you a reality check about your new post-transplant life. Your team psychiatrist is available to listen and advise. You have in your body a foreign organ that used to belong to another. It is normal that there are some issues of identity and integration to work through. Professor Sharp says it is possible that behavior that may be considered unusual may in fact be a natural response to unnatural circumstances. Relax. You really do have the rest of your life!

CHAPTER NINE

Post-Transplant Body Image

Transplantation will not give you the body beautiful; nor will it automatically add weight. What it will do is present you with some physical challenges. You can moderate some of the effects of transplantation's medications, and time will take care of some others. You will have to contend with weight gain, scarring, and excessive hair growth precipitated by the effects of transplant surgery and immunosuppressant drugs. This chapter deals with some ways of coping with these physical changes.

Prednisone has major side effects on the body as well as on the emotions. Even though your dose may be low soon after transplant, and lower until withdrawal, this powerful drug has had time enough to have unpleasant effects.

Have you ever seen an infant on television who has just had an organ transplant? Often there is some drama associated with the child's good fortune, and the event is newsworthy. It is possible that you have thought that there is decidedly something wrong with this child. The cheeks are very puffy, and there is a great deal of hair for one so young, not just on the head but also on the arms and legs, even the eyebrows. Of course. The child is on immunosuppressants. Prednisone, a steroid, and the other antirejection drugs cause degrees of puffiness, weight gain, excessive hair growth, and other side effects. We have discussed the emotional effects of prednisone therapy. In this chapter we discuss the physical side effects.

Weight Gain

Julie R. Ingelfinger, M.D., a coauthor of *Coping with Prednisone,* says of weight gain:

> *Steroid treatment may cause weight gain and redistribution of body fat even if you watch your diet. Some people just do get more side effects than others. But there is a lot that you can do. Steroids do stimulate the appetite, leading to food-eating rampages of monumental proportions for some people. You may be thin, fat, or average in weight when you start steroids. If you are already overweight, going on high-dose steroids can worsen the situation.*

A deceptive phenomenon occurs at transplant. For the first few days after surgery, the recipient has no appetite to speak of. The transplant team, the caregiver, and the family all conspire to get the recipient to eat. Nutrition, especially protein, is necessary for healing. Then, in part because of prednisone, there is a radical reversal and the new recipient can't get enough to eat.

Janet prepares all her patients by telling them that the team will obsess about your eating until you finally get the message. Then your appetite will come back and you will think everything is going well. That's when your coordinator will tell you that you need to watch your weight. Post-transplant eating is probably the most contradictory part of the transplant process. I often dwell on better ways to deal with post-transplant appetite, but I cannot devise a better way to deal with the issue when one is really out of control; once again, it is clear that wellness is the responsibility of the recipient. Observe this exchange from a transplant support group:

"I don't want to be fat anymore! I talked to my primary-care physician yesterday, and he said that even if I am completely weaned off prednisone, the side effects may never go away. He told me not to dwell on it. I found this very difficult to accept."

"I have not lost one single pound. I talked to my nephrologist, and she said that it will be very difficult to get rid of the weight. She also said that most transplant recipients just accept it and stay fat."

"I have been on prednisone for two and a half years. Overall, I have gained about forty pounds. The weight is in the typical prednisone places: face, back of neck, tummy. I have tried everything to lose the weight. Nothing works."

But then there is this response:

I'm a liver transplant recipient—two years out next month—and I certainly haven't accepted the weight gain. During my first year post-transplant, I was on anywhere from 10 to 20 milligrams of prednisone, and, yes, I gained about twenty-five pounds. But as soon as my dosage dropped below 10 milligrams, the weight just started coming off. It isn't easy, but it really does help when the prednisone munchies are gone. I try to walk at least two miles every day at a fairly quick pace, but I have never adjusted my diet. I eat a normal, semi-healthy diet. I am well aware that I have had it easy. A lot of my transplant friends struggle every day with their weight. But take heart—you can win this battle. It just takes time, exercise, patience, and a healthy, well-balanced diet.

David's attempts at post-transplant eating failed miserably. We tried everything to get him to take in the much-needed calories. Immediately after transplant a wave of nausea would come over him when he heard the food cart coming down the hospital hall. He lost over fifty pounds before he could eat and keep food down. His appetite gradually increased, but he vowed that he would never be as heavy as he was prior to transplant. He even went to the extreme of having his suits refitted. Needless to say, he has now bought new, larger suits.

COMBATING THAT WEIGHT GAIN

What can you do about prednisone and weight gain? This last recipient quoted was on the right track. Dr. Ingelfinger prescribed a diet plan for her sister who had an autoimmune disorder and was on prednisone. The diet was low in salt, fat, and simple carbohydrates. Such a diet is low in calories but not in vitamins and minerals. You will have to find the diet that works well for you. Don't go overboard and starve yourself. Ask your team about counseling from a nutritionist or ask your coordinator for a diet that takes all of the post-transplant protocol into consideration.

You were probably on a low-salt diet before transplant. Your taste buds may still react to salt unhappily. Stay on a low-salt diet while you are on prednisone. After all, you are already used to it. I remember that shortly after surgery, while I was still hospitalized, I was allowed some bacon on the hospital tray. I didn't want to eat at all, so for a while, I was allowed anything I wanted. I loved bacon and was looking forward to being able to eat it after so many months of abstinence. But I couldn't tolerate the salty taste. Take advantage of your distaste for salt. It will help keep your weight down.

Exercise is as important as diet. Eugenio, Dr. Ingelfinger's sister, says:

When I was taking prednisone, I sometimes felt like a victim of the cure, instead of like a lucky patient who was taking a miracle drug. Controlling my diet was one way to feel less victimized. Exercising was another effective way to gain a measure of power. Not only did it give me a sense of regaining my strength, but it also made me feel that I was combating some of the potential side effects of prednisone.

Postmenopausal transplant patients are at greatest risk for bone loss, or osteoporosis. It is important that such recipients engage in a regular exercise program, preferably weight-bearing, and take calcium daily. Weight-bearing exercise is best for fighting bone loss. If you think of it, the best exercise is walking—for you are bearing the weight you have gained as you walk! Other good exercises are tennis and weightlifting. Aerobics exercises are good for your general health.

THE EFFECT OF AGE ON WEIGHT GAIN

You read of the recipient who immediately dropped some weight when her prednisone dosage was reduced. Not all will have this experience. Whether you do or not will depend in part on your age. My specialist remarked to me very wisely that I might not feel as energetic after my transplant as I had hoped because I was older—older than before I became ill. Most recipients have been ill a very long time and have really been living on will power. Most have not had much quality of life—especially those on assist devices. Several years may have elapsed before your return to good health through organ transplantation. You may find that you do not get rid of the extra weight easily. You may have to rely once again on self-discipline in order to diet and exercise. The young person and the person who became swiftly and acutely ill may be more energetic than some of us and lose weight more quickly. Still, the rest of us do not want, after undergoing transplant, to end up in jeopardy of dying from obesity! Keep up those good habits you practiced before transplant. Diet and exercise to feel good about yourself. Work on your self-image, and your body image will follow.

Acne

Steroids also cause skin changes, such as acne. This problem can be awfully embarrassing—for adults and children alike. This problem can be treated in much the same way as conventional acne problems. Keep the skin clean and try some of the antiacne products on the market (make sure you consult with your transplant team first). If necessary, consult with a dermatologist (in conjunction with your transplant team). Remember that this problem will only persist for as long as you are on the prednisone.

Scarring

Yes, a pretty bad scar will remain following any transplant procedure. Some may wear it as a badge of honor. Others will only tolerate it at best

WHAT ABOUT TEENS?

If adults have a hard time coping with the effects of transplant, just imagine what it is like for the self-conscious adolescent. To tell adults that their self-image is more important than their body image is one thing; to tell teenagers, who have enormous peer group pressure, is quite another.

Steroids, including prednisone, can cause skin changes, including acne, stretch marks, and redness in the cheeks. The adolescent is already subject to acne and all of the accompanying hormonal changes, including mood swings.

Appearance is everything during adolescence. The side effects we have discussed—weight gain, hair growth, acne, and other skin problems—are a dread to the teenager. In order to avoid the side effects, the adolescent recipient may resist being compliant with taking his or her medicine.

Young patients simply must be active members of their own transplant team. Their cooperation in their own healing is essential. They can control prednisone-induced acne just as they would if the acne were hormonally induced. They can wash the affected areas carefully and consult their coordinators about antiacne medication.

Janet suggests that the relationship between the teenage recipient and the coordinator can actually predict the outcome of the transplanted organ. When the relationship is strong, the teenager can address issues such as self-image, birth control, and recreational drug use with the coordinator much more realistically and openly than with the teenager's parents.

The teenager, just like the adult, can exercise in order to retain muscle tone and bone density. Lifting weights is helpful and socially accepted even for young girls. Walking and other aerobic exercises are very helpful for the adolescent who is still growing.

It is easy for the adolescent to be shortsighted and believe that staying off medication will solve his or her problems. The best way to offset this approach is to explain the nature and necessity of the transplant medication. The teenager must make the regimen his or her own, or he or she will naturally rebel against it, since it has such undesirable side effects. The teen must understand why the medicine is essential.

Another reason for possible noncompliance among adolescents is that most have had little experience with illness other than their own. They associate illness with feeling unwell all of the time. Post-transplant, they may feel well all of the time, so they may assume that they are cured. No more illness means no more medication. On the other hand, if they are experiencing discomfort as a side effect of a medication, their simple solution to the problem is to cease taking medication.

Resisting complying with their medication is also a way that teens may choose to assert their independence. After many years of teaching adolescents and young adults, one day it finally hit me—often (but, of course, not always) youth and immaturity may cause poor judgment. The young person frequently takes in information and some little experience and forms a faulty judgment, on which he or she acts. The caregiver of a post-transplant adolescent has quite a road ahead. It is a road, however, that has its rest stops of joy. Every mother and father prefers its twists and turns to the journey of the weak, fragile child who was theirs before transplant. One mother reports the following:

> *This is a child who seven months ago could not make it up a flight of stairs without assistance; who missed half the school days of the year. Now she ice skates in gym with her class and skips up the steps three at a time to school. She took a sailing vacation for Christmas (very rigorous—like camping afloat) and proudly wore a bikini, displaying her hardearned scars as she leapt off the side of the boat (terrifying her mother). She is planning to go to camp this summer too.*

and may be self-conscious about it. Loved ones know the story that the scar represents and may feel very tender toward it. Are bikinis now out of the question for the young transplant recipient? Well, a lot depends on *your* attitude, not the viewer's.

"Scars seem to be fascinating," says Nichola Rumsey, a coeditor of *Visibly Different: Coping with Disfigurement.* We may understand this assertion better than our immediate ancestors did. After all, we live in the midst of a time when body art, tattooing, body piercing, and even intentional branding and scarring are popular.

The person with a scar is likely to be asked, "What happened to you?" Rumsey suggests that the narrative that follows the question is the person's best means of coping. The story behind the scar is just as important to the healing process as the wound itself. When the scar is visible on the beach, for example, this might be the occasion for a transplant recipient to talk to an acquaintance about the experience of organ transplant and organ donation. We said earlier that you will always be a walking testament to the success of organ transplant. Just don't get carried away and end up with an indecent exposure charge!

The surgical scar, like most scars, will fade with time, but never entirely. You have some control over the extent of scarring by your treatment of the scar after discharge. Certain oils and ointments obscure the outlines of the scar. Coconut oil, applied often and generously, reduces the severity of the surface scar tissue.

Excessive Hair Growth

The problem of excessive hair growth may be more problematic for women than for men. Both cyclosporine and prednisone cause hair growth and do not discriminate about where on the body such growth occurs. It usually occurs in places where one already has body hair. That might mean that one may grow more facial hair than usual. A man can simply grow a beard if he likes or shave it off if he does not like it. A woman, on the other hand, must resort to depilatories, waxing, and frequent leg-shaving. She will be hairy in unwelcome places such as her face and arms. She will have more than enough eyebrow hair. As with all of the side effects we discuss, hair growth decreases as immunosuppressant drug dosages do. This fact is not much comfort for the weeks, even months, of feeling like a werewolf.

Plucking and waxing may be hard on the skin, since prednisone also causes skin sensitivity. These issues vary with the individual. Some may tolerate waxing easily and others not. Skin tissues vary widely. Ask your coordinator about a safe depilatory, one that won't compromise your low tolerance for infection.

I had three facial waxes early in the post-transplant period. I tolerated the procedure well. Since then I have removed facial hair by using a battery-operated hair removal device. It gets at the hair follicle better than tweezers, but it hurts just as waxing does. I remember feeling as though I just couldn't undergo any more pain and discomfort after transplant. So I sometimes alternated the more painful procedures with bleaching, especially in the "moustache" area, the upper lip. I am a brunette—at least I was before I began dying my hair gray. The blondes may have it easier. There are new hair removal solutions on the market. Most of them contain anti-inflammatory agents, so check with your coordinator before use.

Emotional Side Effects
and Your Physical Perception

The excessive hair growth, weight gain, and other unsightly side effects will diminish and are treatable. One problem, though, is that they occur in conjunction with the emotional side effects of the same drugs. We are vulnerable emotionally. We are likely to be self-conscious in the early post-transplant period, and any slight changes can easily affect us. The term "thin-skinned" takes on a whole new meaning!

SELF-IMAGE

Your image of your body is, of course, subjective. How you feel about yourself has everything to do with how you see yourself, even in the mirror. Unfortunately, there may be some truth to the saying that women look in the mirror and see what is wrong, while men look in the mirror and see what is right! Regardless of gender, what others will see is someone who is robust and in good health, in contrast to the frailty you projected before transplant. Enjoy the strength your revived body has after transplant. Your self-image, which is not the same as your body image, needs your attention. If you feel good about yourself, you will look good. Your inner peace and your self-confidence will project a healthy, happy personality. Health and happiness are attractive qualities. You want to feel proud of yourself now more than ever. That good, honorable self-pride will not let you slip into lazy, unhealthy habits again.

Conclusion

Your body image is your perception of your outer self. Your perception may not always conform to reality. It is modified by your emotions and your psychological and social influences. Your self-image—that is, your image of your self-worth—is very much within your control. Of course you can diet and exercise and use soap and water and various oils and ointments. What you cannot do is sit and wait for strength and beauty to return! Your total wellness is your biggest post-transplant job, and it is pretty much all up to you.

CHAPTER TEN

Post-Transplant Lifestyle Issues

As you recover from your transplant, you are most likely anxious to return to life as usual—and for the most part, that is possible and is even encouraged. There are, however, some lifestyle issues you must pay attention to as you move on in your back-to-normal life.

Skin Sensitivity to Sunlight

Transplant drug therapy places the recipient at risk from the rays of the sun. Skin cancer is the most common risk. Prednisone causes thinning of the skin. Even after you are entirely off prednisone you are still at risk for skin cancer. You will be immunosuppressed and therefore at risk for all cancer. Skin cancer is the one you can do most to avoid. In his book, Jim Gleason cites dermatologist Clark C. Otley, M.D., of the Mayo Clinic:

Approximately 35 percent to 70 percent of organ transplant patients develop skin cancer within 20 years following transplant surgery, depending on geographic location. Prior sun damage combined with immunosuppression is a recipe for disaster. We're seeing pa-

tients with hundreds of skin cancers developing per year following transplant surgery. This can ruin a person's quality of life.

You may have the feeling that you are getting conflicting messages from this book. We say live as normally as you can; we imply that walking is a very good exercise post-transplant; and then we tell you that you must be careful out-of-doors and that you are very subject to skin cancer. Well, of course, use the usual precautions that everyone should be taking, including using sunscreen, wearing clothing that leaves little skin exposed, and avoiding being in the sun during the times when ultraviolet rays are strongest—between 11 a.m. and 3 p.m. We spent ten wonderful days in the British Virgin Islands without difficulty by practicing these simple precautions. We had fun in the sun—without the burn! At home again I did not take these admonitions seriously enough. I have lived in Texas all of my life. I have always loved the outdoors and have always been a sun worshiper. I especially love the beach and water. I am not fair, so I assumed that I was invulnerable to sun damage. I have also believed, as so many do, that I look better with a tan. I even go so far as to believe that I look thinner with a tan. Well, this summer I had my first, and I hope my last, basal cell carcinoma removed. I had a mole on my chest, open to the rays of the sun, which turned out to be skin cancer. I have since changed the time of day I spend in the sun. I walk on the beach every day, but at about seven in the evening. It is still beautiful—I am just not getting tan!

Exercise and Sports

As we've been saying throughout this book, exercise before and after transplant is very important, though contact sports should be avoided because of your disposition to bone and muscle loss from prednisone. A gentleman who received his kidney from his son had this to say:

A few months ago, I experienced excruciating pain in my middle spine area attributed to swinging a golf club for the first time in al-

most a year. . . . Lo and behold, I have two compressed (fractured) vertebrae and osteoporosis. They have me on massive doses of vitamin D and calcium and a nasty drug called Fosomax (alendronate sodium). I'm told the condition is caused by the prednisone. I started on 30 milligrams a day and am currently on 7.5 milligrams a day. The head transplant surgeon tells me I probably will be on some amount of prednisone forever. I should also tell you that I'm sixty-three and have always been fit. I've exercised in the gym three to five days a week since I was forty-two. It's not like I am a candidate for osteoporosis anyway.

This reference is meant to be cautionary. Most recipients are withdrawn from prednisone before there is severe bone damage. If the dose has remained high for an extended time, the recipient might ask or be asked to take a bone density test.

Janet recommends that if you have had a history of broken bones or are a woman between the ages of forty and sixty and have been listed for transplant, you ask the transplant team to perform a baseline bone density test prior to transplant. This test will serve as a reference if your post-transplant period is complicated with bone pain. The recipient should also check with the team about the kind and duration of exercise and sports activities you wish to engage in. Contact sports are not recommended, but neither is a sedentary lifestyle. You did not go through transplant to become a couch potato. Common sense will work well for you as you manage your post-transplant life.

"When can I begin exercising?" Janet gets asked this question a lot. You can start walking outside as soon as you are discharged from the hospital, increasing that activity all along. You should probably restrain from jogging for the first six to eight months, but you can fast-walk. Weightlifting should be avoided until after the first year. You want that incision to heal completely. Weightlifting can strain muscles and tear adhesions that can cause hernias in the incision. Nerves are cut during the transplant and cause numbness in your abdomen or chest. You may do more exercises than are good for you and not feel pain, so you may not realize the damage. Riding a bike is a very good exercise once you've built up your stamina and can usually be started about three months post-transplant. When the Transplant Games were held in Texas, a young woman who had had a liver transplant won the 5,000-meter running race just eight months after surgery. Another liver recipient we know took first place in a 5,000-meter bicycle race four months after transplant. David won three silver medals in the same games—two in weightlifting and one in table tennis.

DRIVING POST-TRANSPLANT

Patients who have been sick for a long time with end-stage chronic disease and may not have driven a car for a few years because of their disease or their confusion probably need to practice driving for a while before taking it up again. Some may have had their licenses revoked or have an expired license because they haven't been driving; they may need to take the driving test again. Transplant surgeons are very quick to tell everyone that they can drive six weeks after surgery. I recall one recipient who, after eight weeks, asked the transplant surgeon if she could drive. He replied, "Well, it's been eight weeks, of course you can." Janet got a phone call from her daughter that afternoon; she was horrified, wanting to know why we told her mother she could drive. I said, "It's been eight weeks since surgery." She said, "You don't understand. My mother has never driven a day in her life. She doesn't know how to drive, and now she is insisting that she was told that she could!"

Driving is an issue that should be dealt with very seriously by the coordinator, the recipient, and the family. The family knows more about the history of the recipient's activities before transplant.

TRAVELING POST-TRANSPLANT

When you feel strong enough to travel, you should be able to. I suggest you don't go out of the country until it's been at least a year since your transplant, and then you should be very careful about traveling to underdeveloped countries. Keep in mind that any country that requires that you receive a live vaccine is possibly off limits. Travel to countries that require vaccinations to enter should be discussed with the transplant team before making any travel plans. It is probably wise to speak to your coordinator when you plan to travel. She or he may be able to give you a list of transplant centers in your travel area. Such information can relieve your anxiety about what to do and where to go should there be an emergency. Often your coordinator will know a coordinator for you to contact. She or he will have names and phone numbers.

FLU SHOTS POST-TRANSPLANT

Every transplant recipient should have a flu shot annually. Remember that when an immunosuppressed patient gets the flu, it is a little worse than for someone who is not immunosuppressed. We want to try to avoid those illnesses. One of the problems with your contracting the flu is that any viral infections can cause dehydration. With dehydration, your blood becomes a little thicker, and it is possible that clots may form in your arteries, blocking those arteries that were sewn in at transplant. You should always try to drink plenty of fluids, and get medical attention when you get signs or symptoms of the flu.

OTHER VACCINES POST-TRANSPLANT

As we have said, your transplant team may not allow you to receive any vaccines that contain live viruses after your transplant. For example, you may be applying for a new job where a measles vaccine is required. You may have had the measles as a child, but your resistance is low. Check with your team before taking the measles vaccine or a booster. If you live with a child who has mumps, measles, or chicken pox, stay away from him or her for fourteen days. Avoid children who have received vaccines as part of their school requirements. Children shed viruses from vaccinations in their urine for fourteen days after they are given this live virus, and this circumstance can cause serious infection in immunosuppressed people.

POST-TRANSPLANT CONTACT WITH PETS

Dogs are often good company for recovering transplant recipients. Dogs can, however, spread bacteria that can potentially cause problems for the recipient. Janet suggests that you wash your hands after petting or playing with your dog. Cats are OK as long as you do not change the kitty litter. Airborne bacteria from litter can cost an immunosuppressed recipient his or her life.

Birds can carry exotic bacteria that can be lethal to immunosuppressed patients. Birds have to be housed in a separate room from the new recipient. Remember this advice should you visit a bird sanctuary or the birdhouse at the zoo. A contained, humid bird sanctuary is a dangerous place for the lungs of a recipient to be!

RISKY POST-TRANSPLANT BEHAVIOR

Skydiving, bungee jumping, parachuting, and any high-risk behaviors need to be thoughtfully considered. I can't say that the activity would pose any direct risk to your transplanted organ. I think that you must consider that it has taken a long time, after transplant, to return to the healthy state where you are now—do you want to risk having a problem? High-risk activities are a much bigger risk for immunosuppressed person than for those with average immunity. A broken bone, a laceration, or blunt trauma to the abdomen has the potential to be a life-threatening experience for the transplant recipient. This advice is not to be interpreted as "Don't exercise"! Just choose your activity wisely.

POST-TRANSPLANT HAIR TREATMENTS

Janet says that a lot of older women ask her about hair permanents after transplant. She thinks it better not to get a perm or have your hair dyed for the first six months after transplant. These treatments will not take on the hair immediately post-transplant. It has something to do with prednisone (what doesn't!). The combination of the steroids in the bloodstream and the chemicals in hair dyes and perms nullifies the process. You won't hurt yourself, but you will probably be wasting money. During the few months immediately following transplant, you will notice changes in your hair, especially the texture of it. It would be smart to wait before trying a new look.

SMOKING AFTER TRANSPLANT

Never under any circumstances should a patient smoke post-transplant. The immunosuppressed person is more prone to cancer as it is, without adding to the risk by smoking, a known cause of lung cancer. I can say that every patient I have known who has smoked post-transplant has died within one year from lung cancer. If smoking is a problem for you, seek help to quit smoking prior to transplant rather than risking the consequences after the transplant.

TAKING RECREATIONAL DRUGS AFTER TRANSPLANT

Any kind of recreational drugs could affect your liver, so if you are a liver transplant recipient, this activity is dangerous. Like alcohol, which we discussed earlier, some drugs will interfere with cyclosporine and tacrolimus levels and can put the user at risk for rejection. Recreational drug use should be avoided at all costs post-transplant. Solid organ transplant recipients should avoid all nonsteroidal anti-inflammatory medication, such as ibuprofen (Motrin, Advil, etc.), aspirin, and naproxen sodium (Aleve). These drugs can cause renal failure in the immune-suppressed person.

TOXIC FUMES

Any time you are around toxic paint fumes or other such environmental hazards, you should be very careful not to have extended exposure. You should wear a surgical mask or some kind of protection over your nose and mouth during exposure to prevent any inhalation that might cause an inflammation in the lungs, resulting in pneumonia. These reactions could be lethal in a transplant recipient.

Post-Transplant Social Relations

In the first days or even weeks at home, the recipient will be glad simply to be in familiar surroundings and to rejoice in the presence of family and immediate friends. We have said that you will return home from the hospital more immune suppressed than you will be at a later time. This condition has its social implications. Your caregiver should screen your visitors. That screening will be necessary if your family and friends are not aware of what it means to be immune suppressed and come calling with colds or flu. Even if they know that they have recently been exposed to a virus, they should postpone their visit. This screening will be difficult for everyone, but it is essential. The new recipient is just too vulnerable to any bacteria or viruses. Children, even one's own, are walking contagions. Be careful around them. They are exposed outside the home, when they are in day care or school, to other children's diseases. Ask your adult friends not to bring children to see you for a while and refrain with your own children from usual household contact like sharing a fork or a glass or tasting food.

CROWDS

It is sensible to avoid crowds for a while, especially during the flu season. The same is true for crowded elevators, a doctor's office, a movie theater, a sports event, or church services. If possible, attend an event when there are fewer people present. Wait for a second elevator; find the least crowded waiting room.

Janet recalls that David wanted to go to a baseball game shortly after discharge. Janet wanted to encourage outings but was not thrilled with a stadium full of people as an occasion for one. She called ahead of time and bought tickets that put David in an aisle seat. They arrived at the ballpark an hour before the game began in order to avoid the crowds. After the last out of the ninth inning, they remained in their seats until the crowd dispersed and then exited the ballpark.

You can catch a cold from someone who may not even know that he or she is catching one, so hugs and kisses should be extended with great discretion. I came home from the hospital in late November and made it through the holidays without a sniffle, until a New Year's eve party when, at the stroke of midnight, I kissed a friend who had a cold. My friend should have known better, but then, so should I.

Your team will gradually program your antirejection drugs so that your own immune system will surface a bit and you will have some protection against infection. In the meantime, be careful.

Once a year has passed since your transplant, if you feel well and have no serious setbacks, there is an inclination to feel complacent. Recipients get the feeling that they want to be able to act "normally," to be like everyone else. You can have an insistent urge to return to pretransplant or preillness life. This return might be to lifestyle choices or habits that are not compatible with your transplanted status. We do a disservice to the transplant population if we assume that no one has received a transplant because of a dangerous or abusive lifestyle. A recipient might need to participate in a support group in addition to his or her transplant group. At the same time, he or she may need to avoid some societies or gathering places—like the bar "where everybody knows your name."

Becoming a transplant recipient has presupposed some healthful choices and some lifestyle changes. You would not have been admitted to candidacy had you not pledged, in one credible way or another, to forego some compromising activities. There are those, unfortunately, who, while they are feeling guilty that someone had to die for them to live, at the same time are engaged in habits that threaten their transplant. This behavior puts a whole new spin on "crying in your beer." It makes no sense, after all that you and your loved ones have been through. Enjoy your good health! There are plenty of ways to join in recreation that do not threaten your life or another's.

POST-TRANSPLANT MARITAL RELATIONS

For some couples, illness and the post-transplant period have masked some problems in the marital relationship. After transplant, these issues have to be faced along with those the new life presents. Some of the "new" problems presented include the rush to get back to normal as soon as possible.

One recipient's wife says:

My husband is so much better than he was—I expected him to just be "normal" right away. He is in many ways a different man from the one I married. Both of us have had to adjust to the new person he is. I think in some ways it's been harder on him than on me. For example, he can no longer use his diabetes as a crutch to explain problems away or to justify mistakes.

You might be in a rush to prove yourself, to establish that you are as good as new. If you strike this pose, you may be disappointed. You need time to heal and to adjust to medications that cause perceptible side effects. Some of them may affect your moods, as we have seen discussed, and some may affect your sexual function. You may also have a very different outlook on life, and you may feel frustrated at not knowing exactly what to do with your new-found vision.

With regard to these feelings, the wife of a recipient wrote to the online support group: "This is a natural consequence of being given a second chance, and I think it is a good one. Sometimes it takes awhile to find a niche in which to make a difference, so just give yourselves time to find that niche. Rome wasn't built in a day—don't expect too much of yourselves too soon."

Another recipient wrote:

When I first had my SPK (spleen, pancreas, and kidney) transplant, my coordinators warned me that SPKs had the highest rate of post-transplant divorce of all kinds of transplants in their experience. They said to be sure and look to them for help if problems arose. It is a big adjustment, and I know I feel guilty when I'm not just happy all the time, to have been given this second chance at life. And it definitely takes time to find that new niche—I know, I'm still looking. I have a feeling it's an ongoing process and one my husband and I will be engaging in for a long time.

The recipient may not realize that the partner has gone through a lot of changes too. He or she has been living on the edge of a profound loss for a long time. The partner has probably shut down any thoughts of his or her own needs, including sexual ones. She or he may have borne tantrums, depression, and demands for longer than she knew she could stand it. Her patience with the ill partner probably surprised even her. It would seem that now it is her time, but the recipient is struggling with adjustments to new demands.

Often the recipient's partner has felt shut out and alone much of the time. A prednisone patient says that when someone asked her husband how she was, he replied, "She is nuts." And then he explained that she was taking prednisone, and she was not herself, and he felt very much alone. He added, "She does not want me to have anything to do with it; she does not want me to discuss it with her. Every time I try to discuss it with her, I am slam-banged out of it."

Someone who has been shut out or shut down cannot just reopen like a morning flower. It will take some time and some work to adjust to a new, altogether different marital state. A lot of talking is necessary, and so is consultation with a professional.

The really difficult thing about the early post-transplant period is that it is not static. Chemical changes will go on in the body and in the emotions of the recipient for quite a while after discharge, as medications are withdrawn and perhaps some secondary ones are added as needed.

Post-Transplant Sexual Relations

If a transplant recipient is sexually active and not in a monogamous relationship, he or she should most certainly practice safe sex. In this, as in all issues, recipients must remember that they are immune suppressed. They are very subject to all kinds of infections, whether sexually transmitted or not. On the other hand, the recipient does not pose any greater threat to his partner than the ordinary person might. It is important to speak with your physician about sex. Your physician will probably speak to you about the time he or she supposes that you are well enough to resume sexual relations.

According to our on-line transplant surgeon, Dr. Jeff Punch from the University of Michigan Transplant Program, "Different organ transplants behave differently and require different amounts of immunosuppression, so risk of infectious disease is going to vary markedly. What behaviors are specifically risky for transplant recipients is simply not known."

CONDOMS

Condoms don't prevent diseases that are spread by contact between the skin surrounding the penis and the external genitals: herpes, warts, and crabs. An acute herpes infection in a recently transplanted patient is potentially life-threatening.

ORAL SEX

The risk of contracting most infectious diseases through oral sex is less than through intercourse, but it is still possible, especially if ejaculation occurs and especially if there are any sores or wounds of any sort on either partner. The risk between monogamous partners is minimal, but at least washing with soap and water first is recommended.

FRENCH KISSING

The sharing of saliva is going to expose both individuals to whatever diseases are active in one another, for example colds and other viruses. Other serious diseases can also be spread, including mononucleosis, probably the pervasive cytomegalovirus, and herpes.

COUNSELING

A transplant wife suggests to transplant husbands: "Many of the problems you're experiencing now are due to the transplant and the subsequent change in your lives. A counselor should be able to help the two of you distinguish between the post-transplant problems of adjusting and any underlying problems that were already there in the marriage but were dormant."

Once again, there is reason and cause for a therapist to be on your transplant team. Seek him or her out. These professionals on a transplant team are experienced in the kind of post-transplant marital problems you may face.

IMPOTENCE

Some hypertensive drugs can cause impotence, as can some drugs that stabilize mood swings. Since it will be a long time for energy to return to normal, the recipient may postpone sexual relations until he or she feels energetic. Couple this attitude with a closed emotional state in the partner, and there is a standoff, an impasse. One or both of you must move to reestablish intimacy, even if it is not yet what is hoped for; otherwise the marriage may be in trouble.

Transplant Support Groups

Support groups are a common entity in contemporary society. There seems to be a support group for every concern and every challenge. What these groups offer the person who joins one is exactly what the generic title suggests—support.

A transplant support group is likely to be more practical in its communications than other groups aimed at the psychological or emotional lives of the members. This is not to say that the members do not lend emotional support. They do. Much of the group's agenda, however, is spent exchanging and receiving information about life before and after transplant.

Perhaps because transplant is such a recent medical phenomenon, all of us involved in it are hungry for information. To disseminate information about transplant is, of course, the purpose of this book. As we said in the beginning, knowledge is not only empowering, it is also comforting. None of us likes the unknown.

Jim Gleason, who received a heart transplant, writes:

There seems to be a universal feeling of isolation when you are facing a transplant—despite the presence of family, friends, and professional help. This continues as we come back into the world after a transplant. So many challenges to face. So many new things to learn and adapt to. So alone—at least that is what it seems to you as the recipient.

Usually one of the coordinators of the transplant team leads the support group. She follows the lead of the recipients in setting the agenda. Sometimes there are speakers from outside the center whose work is of interest to the group—for example, a representative of a pharmaceutical company.

Sometimes the content of the meeting arises simply from the questions of the participants. In a small center, the group might include all types of solid organ candidates and recipients. In large centers the group may be organ specific. Sometimes the caregivers meet with the group, and sometimes they have separate meetings where they can air the burdens of being a transplant caregiver.

Probably the greatest emotional support comes from being with one's own. As Jim says, the candidate and the recipient have spent many hours feeling isolated. This kind of aloneness just goes with the territory. No one of us feels capable of conveying our feelings about this experience to another. We may try, but we always fall short. How many times have you said, "I just can't explain it"? You have said this both when you felt scared and when you felt euphoric, when you felt dreadfully alone and when you rejoiced.

Jim's wife asked him what he got out of the meetings.

I tried to explain to her that I learned a lot from the sharings, the presentations, the conversations. I enjoyed the company of others who understand the unique experiences and concerns we shared from our mutual transplant experiences. This is especially true of our common appreciation of the daily gift of life. It is inspiring to meet people who are alive so many years after transplant, despite the many trials they have had to overcome in their unique lives. I found myself feeling very fortunate that I had not gone through many of their experiences. Something that may seem so disastrous in my own life was often put in proper perspective as others shared their life stories.

There is probably a support group at the center where you received your transplant. You may already be a member from your days of candidacy. If, however, there is not a group at your center or you are some distance from your center, you can still get support. Ask your coordinator for help or call your organ procurement organization. Transplant Recipient International Organizations (TRIO) can help also.

A really exhilarating experience is to meet some of your on-line support group friends at the annual U.S. Transplant Games, held in different cities each year—yes, real athletic events for real recipients. That's how healthy we can be.

Returning to Work

Every medical study with which I am familiar cites three coping mechanisms for successful transplant recipients: a sense of humor, a positive attitude, and return to work. Now, "returning to work" need not mean to one's previous job. In our discussion of lifestyle, we mentioned the restriction of avoiding toxic fumes. It may be that your previous work involved hazards to your immunosuppressed condition. David could not return to his previous profession as a fireman because of toxic fumes and the risk of trauma to his transplanted organ. He went back to school and retrained in something he already had a start on as a paramedic: he became a surgical technician. David was in his late forties at that time and was not a lover of textbooks! He also did not want to just sit around and let Janet support them.

If you work behind a desk, that is something you can return to more quickly than if you are a postal carrier. I think this is one of those things that need to be worked out between the transplant team and the recipient. I think the transplant team should encourage the recipient to go back to work, to retrain, or to get some rehabilitation. Candidates need to know up front, before they even go into transplant, that for the most part transplant centers are not willing to grant a medical disability to recipients after a year post-transplant. There may be exceptions for circumstances beyond a recipient's control. I think each recipient should know that they are expected to go back to work.

Jim writes this in his Internet publication: "It continues to be a pleasure to share my recovery with coworkers and so many others after returning to work just four months after surgery. The work continues to be rewarding and fun . . . my energy levels have been more than adequate to support this return to work." Jim admits, however, that his spelling has suffered, and he can't remember names. These problems are medication related. Short-term memory loss is another side effect of prednisone.

Another recipient responded to a discussion about working:

Working either full- or part-time can restore the whole person. It can restore dignity and self-worth to our lives. Life goes on regardless of our medical, financial, or personal situations. If we are capable, we should return to productive activity for several reasons. We owe it to our donor, the medical team, the system, the people on the waiting list, our families, and most of all ourselves.

Lori Noyes, a recipient of kidney-pancreas transplant, had this to say:

Yes, working makes it all seem normal again, doesn't it? . . . My transplant center and nephrologist also consider returning to work a major sign of normalcy after transplant. It took me awhile to come back for physical reasons, and it was tough mentally, though not physically. After about three months, I was back in the old swing of the rat race. I am going to win it this time.

Another recipient who is a private investigator says: "I think that returning to both work and reserves has had a very positive effect on my recovery. If you feel you do not want to go back to work, I feel you should find something constructive to do. Volunteer to speak at different organizations about organ donor awareness . . ."

Still another recipient echoes the call for volunteerism:

More recently I have finally found my "new place" in the scheme of things. I receive wonderful satisfaction for my work ethic lifestyle by contributing, in a very meaningful way, to a major fund-raising program, within the scope of the Canadian Transplant Games Association. I really do agree with others' comments that we need to find ways to be useful.

Probably most people return to work after transplant for much the same reason that they began working in the first place—to earn a living. Working was also a kind of rite of passage to adulthood. Post-transplant, it may be a rite of passage back to normalcy and the land of the living. Work imposes a kind of order in our lives, even a kind of saneness, that is very welcome to a recipient who has felt his or her world upended for some time. Clearly, however, the transplant recipient wants to be and feel useful. Working may be a little like taking one's vital signs. Yes, I'm still living and interacting. I'm working.

What of the debt component—the "I owe" uttered by many recipients? This indebtedness may go the heart of the question of who owns the organs that are transplanted. Certainly, while alive, the person whose they are owns them. Do we harbor a kind of belief that after death the organs belong to the community of humanity? That some organs are assigned to needy recipients and that those fortunate few should "pay back" to the human community from which the organs came by being productive citizens of the world? In other words, there may be an awareness, even if unconscious, that human organs are the world's scarcest and most valuable natural resources. We cannot treat their procuring and their retransplantation lightly. We are under some obligation to trade back something honorable and valuable in return. Hence our labor, on which we have traditionally placed value, becomes symbolic of our wellness and our gratitude.

Conclusion

Believe it or not, either serious lifestyle changes or minor adjustments will become second nature in a short while. Precautions and avoidances that may worry you in the beginning of your post-transplant life will be absorbed naturally into your daily routine. In your efforts to protect your transplant, more often than not, common sense will guide you. For real difficulties in compliance and in dealing with problem behaviors, consult the therapist on your transplant team or one your coordinator recommends. By now you should realize that you are not alone. There is an effective support system in your post-transplant life. Take advantage of it!

Conclusion

This conclusion is an afterword from us to you about your future as a transplant recipient. Your future—you have a future! In the language of *Star Trek*, may you live long and prosper! We will sum up some of the practical implications of living with a transplanted organ and some of the rewards. We will review, for the last time, medications, tests, diet, and exercise. We will refer to information that you can find in a website provided by UNOS, Transplant 101—Life after Transplant.

Medication

You will be taking antirejection medication for the rest of your life unless, as we have said, medical researchers come up with a magic bullet. It is important that you take all of your medications every day and on time. You should talk with your transplant team about anything you don't understand.

HELPFUL HINTS ABOUT MEDICATIONS

- Learn everything you can about your medications, including all the possible side effects.

- Capsules should be swallowed whole and should not be opened until time to take them.
- Keep them in their original containers.
- Some medications should not be taken with grapefruit juice. Check with your team about this.
- Do not take any new medicines before checking with the team, not even over-the-counter drugs.
- Let your transplant team know if you are having trouble paying for your medicines.
- Buy all of your medicines from the same pharmacy if possible. They can keep a profile on you and inform you if a new drug might be harmful.
- Keep an up-to-date list of your meds on your person.
- Check even prescribed drugs from another physician with your transplant team. Don't presume that if a doctor prescribed the medication that it is OK.

MANAGING YOUR MEDICATIONS

- Use a pill box, a fishing tackle box, or small baggies to organize your meds.
- Set an alarm clock or a wristwatch as a reminder to medicate.
- Sort out your meds on a weekly basis, for example, every Sunday afternoon.
- Find some routine reminder for taking your meds, especially those taken twelve hours apart. For example, after breakfast on a work day, and again after dinner, if the two meals are twelve hours apart. Organizing meds around mealtimes is always helpful.
- Keep track of how much medicine you have left in order to reorder in time. Some insurance companies will not let you reorder until a thirty-day period has almost elapsed.
- Be aware of which meds should be taken on an empty stomach and which must be taken with food.

CARRYING MEDS

- Keep medications out of the sun and extreme heat, such as in a car trunk.
- Take extra meds with you when traveling, in case you are detained.
- Don't pack your medicines in your luggage.
- Travel with a letter from your doctor for customs and with the original pharmacy containers, if possible.

NONROUTINE MEDICATIONS

- Ask your transplant team about medications that are not part of your transplant regimen but that you might be prescribed on certain occasions.
- Ordinarily you will be prescribed antibiotics before any dental procedure that is invasive.
- You should get certain vaccines every year, such as flu shots.
- Ask your team about supplement medications such as calcium, vitamins, and minerals.

Post-Transplant Lab Tests

The vampires will still be looking for you post-transplant. (Now you are an initiate; you need to know the code: the vampires are the blood-hungry transplant team who always want a sample from you for some test or other). For a time you will come to the clinic regularly, especially as the team adjusts your medications. The team may ask you to monitor at home for a while your temperature, weight, blood pressure, and pulse rate.

You should notify the team of any dramatic changes.

Be sure to keep your clinic appointments.

Diet

You will probably have fewer dietary restrictions post-transplant than you had before transplant. Consult the nutritionist on the team about a diet that is good for you but allows for your likes and dislikes. No one ever keeps to a diet that entails only sacrifice.

You need proteins for healing and complex carbohydrates for energy. You do not need fats, sugar, or excessive salt for anything.

Exercise

We have explained that lengthy illness and certain medications cause loss of bone density and muscle strength. A kidney recipient, in response to a question on-line about muscle loss, responded:

I've got to say the only cure for the loss of tone/strength in the large muscles is to use them, and use them, and use them some more. Repetition and strength building exercise will help. If possible, you might try consulting a good physical therapist or if you belong to a health club ask for specific exercises that will build strength. It is a slow process, no magic pills.

Another member of the same newsgroup says:

Exercise is something which is almost universally endorsed by transplant centers. The usual warnings about consulting your doctor first apply, but more to assure that the exercise will not put the new organ at risk from injury (boxing might be a good exercise, but I wouldn't recommend it for any transplant recipient). The conventional advice about monitoring the pulse rate must be modified for heart transplant recipients and for people who are on medications that affect the heart rate. It is also important to increase the amount of exercise gradually, especially in recipients who were inactive for a long time because of their disease.

The Transplant Team

The transplant recipient is encouraged to call the transplant team for any problem, at any time, no matter how many years the recipient is away from transplant. Do not hesitate. You have built a trust in the team that time will not erode. They have a vested interest in you. They do not want your organ to fail any more than you do. Keep in touch with them, even when everything is going well. Send a holiday card or a thank-you note on your transplant anniversary. If you maintain some contact, it will not be difficult for you to call with a question, or an emergency, even several years after transplant.

As a coordinator who has followed many a recipient through the long process, Janet says:

> *Often the transplant team is remembered fondly at anniversary dates of transplant, especially when the recipient has received a life-saving organ, a heart, lung, or liver. Many express their gratitude and reflect on the things they have been able to do or see with their extended life, for example, seeing grandchildren born, children married, traveling to places they could never go to because of chronic illness, but mostly they are grateful just for everyday things that they had overlooked and taken for granted before illness set in. I like to ask members of the support group if they have seen the movie* The Color Purple. *In it the two sisters are walking through a field of purple flowers and one comments: "I bet God gets really angry when people walk through a field of purple flowers and don't stop to admire them." These are the things that transplant recipients do regularly: stop and smell the flowers, admire a sunset, or listen to the power of the ocean in a single wave.*

Success Stories

Many recipients echo Janet's sentiments about *The Color Purple*. Often a recipient turns to nature for just the right metaphor. The man whom we have quoted earlier, in answer to his own question, "So what is life like post–heart transplant (three-plus years)?" says:

> *Well, tonight I was under that same moon, and this time I was re-*
> *flecting on my blessing of being alive today to enjoy this beach, and*
> *to share this with my many friends through this note—for you see,*
> *you were all there with me—as I listened to the rolling surf, counted*
> *the stars, I prayed for all of you—candidates waiting, donor fami-*
> *lies I now know as my adopted donor family, fellow recipients, sup-*
> *porters (professional and otherwise)—and my eyes filled with tears*
> *of joy as I visited with you there in the quiet night air.*

A recipient, celebrating his fortieth birthday and his second anniversary of liver transplant, has this to say:

> *Tomorrow is two years since I had my life given back to me. It is hard*
> *to believe it when I look at the pictures in my transplant album, and see*
> *how sick I was, and then look in the mirror, that I am the same person.*
> *In reality, I am not. I know I have changed since then, and am trying*
> *to figure out who I am now. It has been an interesting journey so far.*
> *   I also think about my donor and donor family. I wrote them sev-*
> *eral weeks back, and I know they are receiving my letters, although*
> *I have never heard from them. It is enough that they know who I am,*
> *and that what happened to their teenage son was not a death in*
> *vain. Myself and five other people will be celebrating tomorrow. I*
> *hope that the other recipients have also written to them.*

Lori Noyes, whom we have quoted earlier, sums up her experience this way:

> *If I had to do it over again, or I was writing a book for others going*
> *through this, I would say to them that one should learn all they can*
> *about what is happening to them, their options, and what is involved*
> *in caring for their new gift of life. I would also say that they should*
> *find a source of emotional and physical support before and after the*

transplant. Lastly, I would encourage them all to share their experiences by speaking out about organ donation, write a letter to their donor family, and then . . . go back to work!

Vibrant Health

In reviewing all of the medical proscriptions and prescriptions attendant on organ transplantation, it is necessary for us to keep in mind that all of them together do not make for good health. At least, not all of them alone. Christiane Northrup, M.D., asserts that disease screening does not cause good health. It may inform us that we are, at the time, disease free; being disease free is not the same as being healthy. For the organ recipient, medications, tests, diet, and exercise may help keep the organ from being rejected but alone they do not keep the recipient in vibrant health.

Dr. Northrup's prescription for vibrant health consists of:

- Laughter and a sense of humor
- Sunshine and natural light
- Nutritious food
- Clean air and water
- A fulfilling sex life
- Uplifting relationships
- Outdoor exercise
- A satisfying living and working environment
- Natural sleep and relaxation
- Inspiring music
- Rhythmical dance

We are sure that no one is expected to begin rhythmical dance post-transplant. That attempt might be for some a little bit like the lady who wanted to begin driving after transplant after not having driven before. There is a kind of rhythmical dance that can be performed by our consciousness, however, as we bring aspects of our being into harmony.

Many of the recommendations made in this book are the same as those found in health manuals that call for integration, for a wholistic manner of living that takes into account the splendor of the mind and the body as one, in one rhythmical dance. Post-transplant, you may have your first best go at fullness of health. You are aware now of what that means and how it can be attained.

The recipient who wrote about exercise also had this to say:

Many people believe that being immune suppressed means you feel sort of sick and weak most of the time. In my experience, the problem is the opposite: you feel so healthy that you forget that you are immune suppressed and neglect the basic hygiene precautions that are still necessary. So exercise and make yourself strong, but keep washing your hands and stay away from people with active infections.

We began this chapter with *Star Trek*. We end similarly with every good wish for you in your full post-transplant life. "Let's see what's out there." Come back and tell us, if you have the time.

Glossary

Abdominal drain. A plastic tube that allows blood, serum, and bile to exit the peritoneal cavity without difficulty.

Acetaminophen. A mild over-the-counter painkiller that, if used for an extended period or in large doses, may cause kidney or liver failure.

Actigall. See UROSODIOL.

Acute. Referring to a disorder that happens suddenly and is usually of limited duration; often used to describe an organ rejection episode that can be managed through an adjustment in medication.

Amantadine (Symmetrel). An ANTIVIRAL AGENT.

ANA. Antinuclear antibody—evidence that the body has been fooled and is attacking itself, including the liver, in autoimmune disease.

Analgesic. A medication, such as acetaminophen, commonly used to block mild pain.

Anemia. An imbalance in the amount of oxygen carried in the red blood cells.

Angina. Chest pain due to a lack of oxygen to the heart muscle.

Anorexia. A severe loss of appetite.

Antibacterial agent. A medication used to treat or prevent infection with bacteria. An antibiotic.

Antibody. A protein in the immune system that normally attacks anything foreign in the body.

Antifungal medications. Treatment for fungal infections such as candidiasis and cryptococcal meningitis.

Antigen. Anything foreign to the body.

Antihypertensive medications. Treatments for high blood pressure.

Antirejection drugs. Drugs that prevent the body's attack on the new organ.

Antiviral agent. A medication used to combat virus, used especially with hepatitic C infection.

Arrythmia. An abnormal heart rate, either faster or slower than normal, commonly caused by coronary heart disease.

Arteriogram. An x-ray of an artery.

Artery. That part of the circulatory system that carries blood away from the heart.

Ascites. Water retention in the abdominal area; the kidneys become confused and do not excrete the sodium and water that they should.

Assist device. Any number of mechanical devices used to aid in normal bodily functions. For example, a dialysis machine may be required to cleanse the blood of impurities prior to transplant.

Autoimmune disorder. Any condition in which the body's immune system attacks its own tissue.

Azathioprine (Imurox). An immunosuppressant drug.

Bactrim. An antibacterial agent. See SMZ/TMP.

Bile. A product of the liver formed from broken-down red blood cells, it functions as a detergent in the absorption of fat from one's diet.

Bile duct. A duct or tube leading from the liver to the gallbladder and small intestine.

Biliary atresia. Congenital inflammation and obstruction of the bile ducts in the liver, often seen in newborns.

Biopsy. A method by which a tissue sample is obtained with a needle for analysis.

Brain death. When the brain ceases in all its functions. Other parts of the body may continue to function with the aid of assist devices rather than as an operational response to brain function.

Bronchitis. Inflammation of the airways that results in a chronic sputum-producing cough.

Bypass. In transplant surgery, a procedure performed in order to return blood from the lower half of the body to the heart.

Cadaver. A dead body. This term may refer to a body that is brain dead but whose functions are continued by mechanical means until the organs can be recovered.

Candidate. A patient in need of organ transplant.

Cardiac. Referring to the heart.

Cardiologist. A heart specialist.

Cardiomyopathy. A disease of the heart muscle causing a reduction in the strength of the heart's contractions, thus decreasing blood circulation.

Catheter. A tube placed in the bladder to drain urine.

CBC (Complete blood count). An assessment of all of the cellular components of the blood.

CellCept. See MYCOPHENOLATE MOFETEL.

Cholestasis. Inflammation (congestion) in and around the gallbladder, usually associated with right-upper quadrant pain, nausea, and vomiting.

Cirrhosis. Chronic disorder of the liver, marked by inflammation and scarring, which disrupts normal liver function.

Congenital disorders. Birth defects.

Congestive heart failure. A buildup of fluid around the heart that reduces the heart's ability to pump blood.

Contraindication. Problems arising in the screening process that may prohibit a person from becoming a transplant candidate.

Coronary artery disease. A disease of the blood vessel that carries blood away from the left ventricle of the heart through the aorta.

Crohn's disease. A painful gastrointestinal illness of unknown cause that results in fever, diarrhea, weight loss, and deep ulcers in the intestinal tract.

CT/CAT scan. Computerized axial tomographic scan. This technique uses both a computer and x-ray, which, in combination, provide a cross-sectional image of the tissue or body being examined.

Cyclosporine (Neoral, Sandimmune, SangCya). An immunosuppressant drug used to prevent the body from rejecting a new organ.

Cystic fibrosis. An inherited disease that usually appears in early childhood and results in lung dysfunction and an inability of the body to absorb nutrients.

Cytomegalovirus (CMV). A viral infection that causes pneumonia or hepatitis.

Cytovene. See GANCICLOVIR.

Deltasone. See PREDNISONE.

Diabetes mellitus. Commonly referred to simply as diabetes, this disorder results in an abnormally high level of glucose in the bloodstream. It is a pancreatic dysfunction usually controlled by diet or insulin in its milder stages.

Dialysis. An assist process by which an imbalance of chemicals and wastes are mechanically removed from the body.

Diuretic. Type of medication prescribed to lessen water retention; excess fluids are expelled through the kidneys.

Donor–recipient compatibility. A measure of organ matches, either by blood type, tissue, size, or in combination, depending on the specific organ being transplanted.

Dopamine. A blood-vessel constrictor naturally produced by the brain, but also produced synthetically and given intravenously to patients who need blood-pressure support. At low doses, it can help the kidneys produce urine.

Dyspnea. Difficulty in breathing.

Echocardiogram. A procedure used to obtain an image of the heart through the use of sound waves.

Edema. Swelling due to fluid retention.

Electrocardiogram. A tracing that shows the electrical conductivity of the heart.

Emphysema. A disease that damages tiny air sacs in the lungs and results in difficulty in breathing, life-threatening respiratory problems, or heart failure.

Encephalopathy. Mental confusion due to toxins in the bloodstream.

Endoscopy. A procedure in which a tube with a light and video camera is inserted through the mouth and intestines in order to diagnose visually. This procedure is common in the case of suspected ruptured VARICES. Tissue can be cauterized or injected during this procedure when necessary.

FK506. An immunosuppressant drug; see TACROLIMUS, PROGRAF.

Fluoxetine (Prozac). A medication used to treat depression.

Furosemide. A DIURETIC.

Ganciclovir (Cytovene). An ANTIVIRAL AGENT.

Gastroenterologist. A physician who has a broad specialization in the digestive system, including the stomach, liver, intestines, kidneys, pancreas, and gallbladder.

Gingival hypertrophy. A gum disease common among transplant recipients, usually treated with good dental hygiene and plaque removal.

Glomular filtration rate (GFR). A measure of kidney function.

Glucose. A simple sugar in the bloodstream that is largely responsible for the body's energy.

Graft. An organ or tissue transplant.

Heart. The muscular organ that pumps blood to and receives blood from the rest of the body.

Hematocrit. A test used to determine the number of blood cells in a given volume of blood.

Hemochromatosis. Abnormal processing and storage of iron by the body.

Hemodialysis. A regularly scheduled treatment used to cleanse a kidney patient's blood.

Hemoglobin. The element in the blood that carries oxygen to the rest of the body.

Hepatic. Related to the liver.

Hepatitis. Inflammation of the liver coupled with cell damage. The three most common types of viral hepatitis are A, B, and C (once known as non-A, non-B).

Hepatologist. A physician who has specialized in the study of the liver and its diseases.

Hormone. A chemical produced by the glands and secreted into the bloodstream that affects the function of other organs and cells.

Human leukocyte antigens (HLAs). Groups of tissue types used in matching kidneys and pancreases.

Hyperglycemia. A condition in which the glucose (sugar) in the blood is at an abnormally high level.

Hypertension. High blood pressure.

Hypoalbuminemia. Low protein levels in the blood.

Hypoglycemia. A condition in which the glucose (sugar) in the blood is at an abnormally low level.

Hypotension. Low blood pressure.

Ibuprofen. An over-the-counter anti-inflammatory drug used in the treatment of headaches, toothaches, menstrual discomforts, or other relatively mild pains.

Immunosuppression. Prohibiting the body's immune system from attacking a new organ. Immunosuppression is achieved through drugs immediately following transplant and is continued throughout the recipient's life.

Imuran. See AZATHIOPRINE.

Indication. Reasons for signs and symptoms that make one eligible for transplant.

Insulin. A natural hormone produced as a function of the pancreas. It serves as a regulator of glucose (sugar) in the bloodstream.

Internist. A physician who has specialized in diseases affecting internal organs.

Intravenous therapy. Medical treatment given to a patient through a tube into a vein.

Intubation. The use of a breathing tube inserted through the mouth and extending into the lungs.

Islet cells. The cells in the pancreas that secrete insulin and glucogen.

Kidney. The organ that filters and removes waste, toxins, and excess water from the bloodstream as urine. Each of us normally has two kidneys that function in parallel. If one kidney is removed, the remaining kidney will develop the capacity to take over the job of both. The kidney will stabilize, and the body will function normally.

Lactulose. A drug that softens the feces, acts as a laxative, and helps to eliminate toxins otherwise absorbed from the colon into the bloodstream.

Laparoscopy. Insertion of a scope into the abdomen through an incision to view the internal organs.

Laparotomy. An operation involving opening the abdominal cavity, which enables the physician to view the liver.

Lasix. See FUROSEMIDE.

Live virus vaccine. A minuscule dosage of a living virus, which, when introduced into the bloodstream, causes the immune system to react by fighting the virus and "standing guard" against future attacks of the virus or bacteria. In a transplant recipient, the introduction of such a vaccine could be deadly because the immune system has been compromised. Live virus vaccines include those for measles, chickenpox, mumps, rubella, yellow fever, polio, and hepatitis B. Transplant recipients should avoid entering countries in which these vaccines are required.

Liver. The largest of the body's organs; serves as a regulator, monitoring blood and necessary chemicals needed by the rest of the body and dispelling the rest. Unlike the case of the kidneys, we have only one liver. It is considered one of the body's most important organs.

Living related donor. A family member whose organ matches specific requirements for transplantation and who donates an organ or portion of an organ for transplantation.

Living unrelated donor. A non–family member whose organ matches specific requirements for transplantation and who donates an organ or portion of an organ for transplantation.

Living will. A legal document defining your wishes regarding extraordinary life support should there be complications during your illness or during transplant surgery.

Magnesium oxide. A magnesium replacement medication.

Malignancy. A tumor that will continue to grow, eventually affecting other parts of the body. It can result in death if left untreated.

Marginal donor. An organ donor whose organs may or may not be acceptable for transplant. Not every organ that is donated is healthy enough for transplant, as the result of lacerations in the case of a car accident, for example, or perhaps because of the age or lifestyle of the donor.

Multisystem organ failure. When more than one organ is failing and the transplantation of one organ will not improve the function of another.

Mycophenolate mofetel (Cell Cept). An immunosuppressant drug.

Mycostatin. See NYSTATIN.

Neoral. See CYCLOSPORINE.

Nephrologist. A kidney specialist.

Noncompliance. A candidate or recipient's deviation from medically prescribed directives in either lifestyle or dosage of medications.

Nonheartbeating donor. Someone who has died as a result of the termination of life-support systems and who has donated his/her organs.

Nystatin (Mycostatin). An ANTIFUNGAL MEDICATION.

Organ procurement organization (OPO). A regionally governed center that facilitates organ distribution in a given area (see also UNOS).

Orthotopic transplant. An organ graft in which the new organ is placed exactly where the old one was.

Palpitation. Faster- or harder-than-normal heartbeat.

Pancreas. A gland that assists the digestive system, breaking down carbohydrates and protein, and secretes insulin and glucogen.

Paracentesis. A process to remove/withdraw excess fluid from the peritoneal cavity using a needle. It is a quick and relatively easy process, and only a local anesthetic is necessary.

Pericarditis. An inflammation of the tissue around the heart, which may result in chest pain and a buildup of fluid restricting the heart's functions.

Peripheral edema. Swelling of the extremities, such as legs and arms.

Peripheral neuropathy. An inflammation of the nerves resulting in numbness, tingling, or pain in the extremities.

Peritoneal dialysis. A method of assisting the kidneys in ridding the body of impurities, using a catheter, which is inserted into the wall of the abdominal cavity.

Pleural effusion. The collection of fluid around the lungs.

Pneumonia. An infection that causes inflammation of the lungs.

Polycystic kidney disease. An inherited disorder in which cysts develop in the kidneys and ultimately may invade other organs.

Portal vein hypertension. Increased pressure in the veins around the liver and intestines.

Power of attorney. A legal document transferring the power over your financial matters to another person in the event that you become incapacitated.

Pravachol. See PRAVASTATIN.

Pravastatin (Pravachol). Medication used to lower cholesterol and triglyceride levels.

Prednisone (Deltasone). A steroid used after transplant to prevent rejection of the new organ. Like CYCLOSPORINE, this drug has possible serious side effects, but it is essential to life for the transplant recipient.

Primary liver tumors. Tumors in the liver that originate in the liver rather than spread to the liver from another organ, as happens with SECONDARY LIVER TUMORS.

Procurement. Recovering or retrieving an organ for transplantation.

Prognosis. A physician's estimate of the ultimate progression and outcome of a disease.

Prograf. See TACROLIMUS.

Prophylactic. A preventative medication taken to combat opportunistic bacteria, viruses, and fungi.

Prozac. See FLUOXETINE.

Psychotherapy. Therapy to assist patients in coping with psychological pitfalls, such as stress or depression, that could negatively affect the transplant process.

Pulmonary edema. Collection of fluid in the lungs.

Pulmonary fibrosis. Scarring of lung tissue that diminishes the capacity of the lungs to function properly.

Pulmonary hypertension. The inability of blood to flow adequately through the arteries in the lungs. The result is an increase in the blood pressure of those arteries.

Pulmonologist. A lung specialist.

Recovered organ. An organ removed from the donor's body.

Red blood cells. That element of blood that absorbs oxygen and delivers/releases it to the body tissue.

Rejection. Adverse reaction of the body to a new organ, in which it recognizes the new organ as foreign and attacks it.

Renal. Referring to the kidney.

Renal failure. The inability of the kidneys to function properly in removing chemicals and waste from the bloodstream.

Renal replacement therapy. A kidney transplant.

Resection. The removal of the diseased or dysfunctional organ.

Sandimmune. See CYCLOSPORINE.

SangCya. See CYCLOSPORINE.

Sclerosing cholangitis. A narrowing of the liver's bile ducts.

Secondary liver tumors. Tumors in the liver that began elsewhere in the body and have spread to the liver.

Shunt. A tube surgically inserted for the purpose of drainage of excess fluids or for easy access to the bloodstream. There is a high mortality rate associated with this procedure.

SMZ/TMP (Bactrim). Sulfamethoxazole and trimethoprin. An ANTIBACTERIAL AGENT.

Sputum. Mucus produced from a cough.

Steroids. Drugs used in transplantation to inhibit the immune system's attack on the new organ.

Symmetrel. See AMANTADINE.

Synthetic interferon. A drug used to treat hepatitis C.

Systemic infection. An infection found throughout the entire system.

Tacrolimus (FK506, Prograf). An immunosuppressant drug.

Thrombosis. A condition in which the blood clots in the arteries.

Tissue compatibility. An acceptable match, determined by a blood test, between a potential donor and a recipient of kidney, pancreas, or heart transplantation.

T-cell lymphocyte. A type of white blood cell.

Triglycerides. Fat in the bloodstream.

T-tube. A tube placed in the bile duct in order to drain bile into a small pouch outside the body. It is shaped like a T with the tail of the T visible from the outside of the body. The top of the T is positioned in the bile duct.

Tuberculosis. An airborne infection that most commonly affects the lungs and that results in plural effusion and pneumothorax. This infection can be carried by the bloodstream to other parts of the body.

Ultrasound. A method of diagnosing a liver or kidney condition using sound waves.

United Network for Organ Sharing (UNOS). A nonprofit, federally funded private organization that accounts for organs and their distribution throughout the country. This "mother company" maintains the national database, which in turn is accessed by OPOs.

Urea. Protein filtered and eliminated by the kidneys in a healthy body.

Urosodial (Actigall). Medication used to assist the body in thinning the bile and preventing cholestasis in the liver.

Vancomycin. An antibiotic used to treat staph infections.

Varices. Enlarged veins (similar to varicose veins) that develop in the lower esophagus and stomach. They can also present as hemorrhoids.

Ventilator. An assist device used to help patients breathe.

Ventricle. A section or chamber of the heart that pumps blood to the rest of the body.

Wilson's disease. An inherited disorder in which copper accumulates in the liver and nervous system.

Xenograft. An organ or tissue recovered from an animal for the purpose of transplantation into a human.

Index

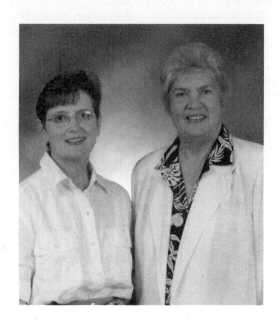

ABOUT THE AUTHORS

ELIZABETH PARR, PH.D. (right), is a professor of English at the University of St. Thomas in Houston. She received a liver transplant in 1994 and has since become an expert on the subject of organ transplantation: she wrote a book and a doctoral dissertation about her experience, and frequently lectures to medical and lay audiences on the topic. Parr lives in Galveston, Texas.

JANET MIZE, R.N., is a nurse transplant coordinator at the University of California, Irvine, transplant program. She, too, is a frequent lecturer on the subject of organ transplantation. President of the International Transplant Nurses Society, she lives in Tustin, California.